Purify Your System for
Health & Beauty

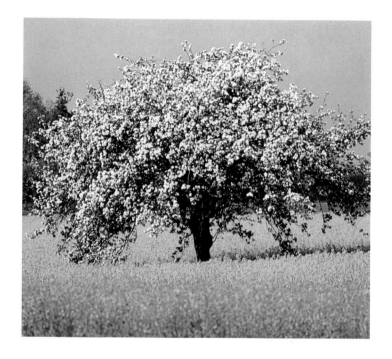

Margot Hellmiss & Falk Scheithauer

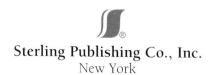

Sterling Publishing Co., Inc.
New York

Library of Congress
Cataloging-in-Publication Data
Available

10 9 8 7 6 5 4 3 2 1

Published 1998 by Sterling
   Publishing Company, Inc.
   387 Park Avenue South,
   New York, N.Y. 10016
Originally published and © 1996 in
   Germany by Sudwest Verlag
   under the title *Gesund und schön
   durch Entschlackung*
English translation © 1998 by
   Sterling Publishing Co., Inc.
Distributed in Canada by Sterling
   Publishing
   % Canadian Manda Group,
   One Atlantic Avenue, Suite 105
   Toronto, Ontario, Canada M6K 3E7
Distributed in Great Britain and
   Europe by Cassell PLC
   Wellington House, 125 Strand,
   London WC2R 0BB, England
Distributed in Australia by
   Capricorn Link (Australia) Pty Ltd.
   P.O. Box 6651, Baulkham Hills,
   Business Centre, NSW 2153,
   Australia
*Manufactured in the United States of
   America*
All rights reserved

Sterling ISBN 0-8069-4219-3

Contents

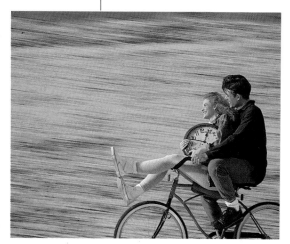

A week of detoxification should be planned in a sensible manner.

Foreword

The Big Spring Cleaning

In just about every household the big spring cleaning takes place when the first days of spring arrive. Windows are washed, carpets are cleaned, upholstery and pillows are carried outside, and doors are opened widely to let the spring sunshine flood the freshly cleaned rooms.

Hallmarks of Winter

Not only did our homes gather dust during the dark time of the year. For most of us, winter didn't pass without leaving its marks. Not enough physical activities, artificial lighting, dry air from heaters, and too many heavy meals were the hallmarks of the cold season. Digestive problems may have occurred—and because of the generally slowed-down pace during the dark days, occasionally circulatory problems may have set in, too. Lazy bowel syndrome also is a common occurrence during the winter, so many metabolic deposits that had formed in the body may not have been eliminated, but stored in the blood and in tissue.

A Healthful Start into Spring

Now, after the winter, the intestines should be unburdened, the organs of elimination should be cleansed, the skin should be exposed to plenty of fresh air, and, via the lungs, oxygen should be pumped into the blood. The beginning of spring is the ideal time of year for an overall tune-up with the aid of a detoxifying or purifying cure.

Not only is the house cleaned traditionally in spring, but your body should be given a spring cleaning too.

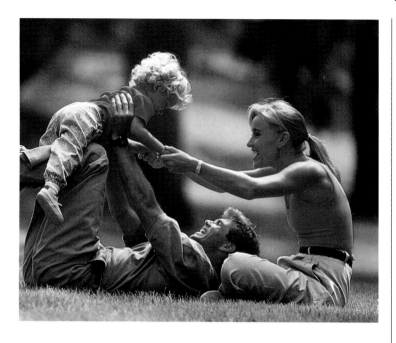

Celebrate the season with a spring cure! You will feel fresh and revived.

Revitalized Through Detoxification

Your meals should be leaner now and enriched by fresh fruits and vegetables and vital substances. This will purge the body of acids and deposits and reduce your weight. With the aid of medicinal plants, breathing techniques, a targeted stimulation of the kidneys, skin care, and many other measures, the detoxification systems of the body can be induced to rid the organism of deposits and toxins. This is done best during a week of detoxification. Thus cleansed, you will feel full of energy, fresh, and revitalized at the beginning of the new season.

Of course, you don't have to plan your week of detoxification or a single day of purification exclusively in the spring. The right time for a spring cure actually can be any time during the year.

Develop a feeling for spring. After a detoxification cure, you will be fit for spring and feel reborn. In this book, you will find many tips for natural and healthful detoxification cures.

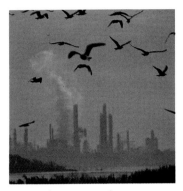

Industry is producing greater quantities of toxins, further polluting the air we breathe.

Technical advancement is destroying more and more of the environment. Even seals living in the far-off northern Arctic Ocean are affected by environmental pollution. This is why we can't avoid facing the problems of the environment.

What Is a Clogged System?

Protect Your Inner Environment— a Commandment of Our Time

Technical advancement seems to go hand in hand with environmental pollution. Throughout the world, there is hardly a spot where the traces of environmental toxins cannot be found. Take the case of the seals living in the northern Arctic Ocean. In the tissue of these animals, highly toxic PCB (polychlorinated biphenyl) was discovered.

The Problems of Increased Population

According to data furnished by from UNESCO, world population has doubled over the last 35 years, increasing to about 5.75 billion. As a result of so many people having to be provided for, the amount of toxins in the environment has hit levels never reached before.

Industry and transportation systems producing billions and billions of tons of pollution (nitric oxide, carbon monoxide, benzene, and so forth) have increased immensely over the last hundred years, burdening worldwide the air we breathe. Agribusinesses producing ever-increasing amounts of food use huge quantities of poisonous pesticides and insecticides, which now can be found in our food and drinking water.

More Than 70,000 Environmental Toxins!

There are currently more than 70,000 toxins in the environment. Among them are such extremely toxic substances as the metals lead, cadmium, and mercury, which mainly enter our food by way of industrial air pollution and water, and substances like acrylic nitrile and PCB (polychlorinated biphenyl). Acrylic nitrile is used in the manufacturing of textiles. PCB, used years ago in textile manufacturing and now more or less banned there, can still be found in food and human breast milk.

As can be seen from these examples, environmental toxins immediately affect everybody. All of us take in such toxic substances with our food, the water we drink, the air we breathe, or by means of skin contact.

Inner and Outer Environmental Protection

The human body has to process every poison it takes in. If this becomes impossible because the organs of detoxification are overburdened, then diseases and even death will occur. Thus, it is a commandment of our time to not only practice "outer" environmental protection, but "inner" as well.

If the organs of detoxification are overburdened, the organism will become diseased. The remedy then is to practice "inner environmental protection."

Insidious Poisoning

Not all the results of this insidious poisoning have been studied so far. Of all the 70,000 environmental toxins, only about 10 percent (7,000) have been examined for their cancer-inducing properties. How the others affect the human organism, especially in the long run, is still unknown—except for a general increase in allergic skin disorders and illnesses affecting the breathing passages.

How to Practice Inner Environmental Protection

Inner environmental protection means reducing our intake of toxins, which we can do, for example, by consciously selecting the food we eat. Because, in the long run, none of us can totally avoid environmental toxins, it is even more important to use measures of detoxification to help the body cleanse itself.

"Man is a healthy [being] who daily destroys his capital of life." (Dr. Max Bircher-Brenner, physician and lifestyle reformer, 1867–1939)

Food Coloring That Can Produce Allergic Reactions

NAME	IDENTIFICATION	OFTEN CONTAINED IN
Tartrazine	E 102	Fizz powder, mustard, syrup, sweets, artificial honey
Chinoline yellow	E 104	Instant pudding, egg coloring, fizz powder
Yellow orange S	E 110	Chocolate-mix drinks, instant soups, marzipan, instant pudding, apricot marmalade, orange biscuits
Carmine	E 120	Marmalades, alcoholic beverages
Ado rubin	E 122	Bread crumbs, brown gravies, instant soups, sweets, biscuits
Amaranth	E 123	Liqueur, ice cream
Cochineal red	E 124	Artificial salmon, fruit jellies, sweets
Erythrosine	E 127	Canned fruit, ice cream
Brilliant black	E 151	licorice, gravies, sweets, artificial caviar
Bixin	E 160 b	Margarine, bonbons

Residues of Metabolism

People who are still using coal-burning stoves are familiar with the grayish-black, hard, and porous little clumps that over time collect on the grate. These are residues of combustion, called slag, which have been compared to certain residues and waste products generated by our metabolism.

Increased Waste in the Intestines

The above image is fitting, because when waste products increase in the intestines, the process of digestion is frequently called combustion. As with "real" combustion, here too waste products are generated. But from the medical point of view, such waste products only can be compared to slag if their transportation is hindered. However, due to a long time of faulty nutrition or overeating, for example, stubborn deposits can form on the walls of the intestines. Such food residues become toxic over the years, and can burden the entire organism.

"It is extremely difficult to convince people that an evil is evil." (George Bernard Shaw, British-Irish writer, 1856–1950)

Where Deposits Are Found in the Body

Not only can these deposits form in the alimentary tract, but they also can occur in the blood, in muscles, joints, and actually in all tissues on the transit route between the blood and the cells of the body.

Deposits that are harmful to our health are urea, uric acid, ammonia, carbon monoxide, lactic acid, ketonic acid, phenol, indole, and skatole, as well as precursors of these materials, called intermediary products.

Toxins

From Without and Within

The environmental toxins taken into our body through the air we breathe or otherwise are not regarded as deposits because they are not products of metabolism nor generated within the body. However, these distinctions between toxins taken in from the outside and toxins generated within the body can be ignored unless it is a matter of acute poisoning.

Toxins taken in from the outside have to be eliminated just like poisons generated by the body. The mechanisms of elimination are more or less the same in this process as long as the insecticide DDT or mercury has not been lodged in the fatty tissue. It is still not clear whether or not in the latter case it can be eliminated at all.

Increased Deposits

It should be added that an excessive intake of toxins will increase the formation of deposits, because the organs of elimination can be overburdened by the onslaught of toxins, which will in turn make the elimination of body-generated deposits more difficult. The toxins themselves can be compared to a kind of slag if their elimination is being impeded and they, literally, clog up the body's pathways of elimination and generally make them less passable. Furthermore, some of the body-generated wastes are pure toxins themselves. This is especially true of phenol, indole, skatole, and fusel alcohol, which are formed during the digestive process and occur in higher concentrations in cases of clogged intestines.

"All things are poisons and nothing is without poison. It is only the small doses that make a thing no longer a poison." (Paracelsus, scientist and physician, 1494–1541)

The Overburdened Transit Route

The billions of cells in the body are not directly provided for by the blood, but by the fluid within the connective tissue. This fluid connects the cells with the blood vessels. Everything that the cells need, like nutrients or oxygen, runs through this fluid. The fluid moves along a transit route, whereby the cells are not only being provided for but are also cleansed. All waste materials from cell regeneration or metabolism are transported by means of the transit route.

What Will Happen If the Transit Route Is Jammed?

If you eat too much protein (meat, eggs, cheese, and so forth), for example, cells satiated from former meals cannot take in the arriving nutrients. These nutrients then remain on the transit route. Too much protein is acid-forming, so the fluid of the connective tissue will become overly acidic. It will thicken and be less able to supply the cells with vital substances, like oxygen or minerals.

Consuming too much alcohol, black coffee, or sweets also can produce too much acid and in turn an increase in deposits. The transit route will become an area of blockage (called mesenchyme blockage) for materials that should have been eliminated a long time ago. Because the fluid of the connective tissues surrounds every cell in the body, the whole organism will be affected. The continuous blockage of the transit route is the primary cause for gout, rheumatism, and arteriosclerosis (calcification of the arteries), as well as lowered immunity, depression, bronchitis, fistula, boils, and other ailments.

All diseases have a single underlying cause: the contamination of body fluids. (motto of naturopathic medicine)

Poor Blood Circulation

In our general latitudes, every second death can be traced to heart and circulatory diseases. For a comparison, only every fourth person dies of cancer. One of the primary causes of the failure of the heart and circulation—aside from organic disorders such as congenital heart disease—has to do with a poor flow of blood. This can be traced in most cases to a thickening of the blood and/or a blockage of the arteries (arteriosclerosis). Both cause the blood to flow poorly or not at all in a certain area of the body. Organs, muscles, tissues, and so forth will only be provided for poorly or might even be destroyed.

The signs of the onset of a hardening of the arteries are easy to overlook. But every second death in Western countries can be traced to diseases of the heart and circulatory system.

Intimations of Future Problems

In the beginning stages of poor circulation, the effects might not be felt dramatically. The finest branches of the arteries, the blood capillaries, are so thin that together they have a length of about 100,000 kilometers (or 62,000 miles). In the beginning, disturbances of the blood flow within the capillaries will cause only slight trouble. But this trouble indicates quite alarmingly that the problem with blood flow is starting to worsen. Perhaps, some time in the future, in the area of the larg-

Signs Indicating the Onset of a Hardening of the Arteries

➤ Tingling in fingers or toes

➤ Feelings of numbness

➤ Cold hands or feet

➤ Extremely pale skin

➤ Arms and/or legs frequently falling asleep

➤ Difficulty concentrating

➤ Forgetfulness

er arteries, more threatening incidences might occur that eventually will lead to a stroke or heart attack.

Preventing Arteriosclerosis

Preventive measures you can take are the following:
➤ Fasting
➤ Diets without animal fat and added salt

Eating less eliminates deposits in the blood vessels and improves the blood flow. Furthermore, the harmful substances of cholesterol, the LDL (low-density lipoprotein), will be reduced.

According to the latest findings, folic acid in particular

People who smoke a lot risk not only lung cancer but also circulatory problems, a stroke, and a heart attack. They are systematically poisoning their entire body.

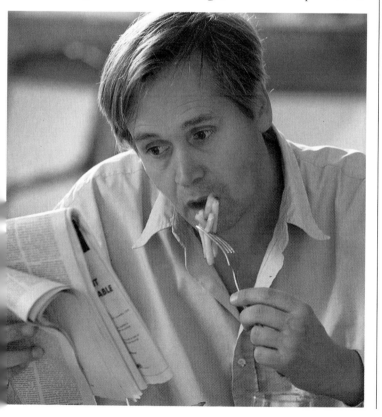

Eating fast foods hastily and frequently consuming soft drinks loaded with sugar will increase deposits, possibly leading to circulatory problems.

seems to prevent arteriosclerosis. Folic acid is found, for example, in spinach, broccoli, asparagus, and red beets.

Pain in Muscles and Joints

An indication of deposits in the muscle tissue is painful tension in the shoulder or the neck. Pain in the muscles, known as myalgia, is partly due to deposits. Myalgia arises if lactic acid produced during physical activity is blocked and thus not eliminated correctly. The muscle tries to rid itself of the fluid and presses into the area of the nerves, which leads to pain and can later produce neuritis or even sciatica. If hyperacidity of the tissue continues for a long time, joints and especially cartilage can be affected. This is one of the causes of rheumatoid arthritis.

Myalgia is a common manifestation of deposits. After physical exertion, the lactic acid in the muscle tissue is only dismantled slowly.

A Health Checklist

The following questions will help you determine easily whether or not you should undertake a purification cure. If you answer "yes" to only a single question, purifying your system would be advantageous for you.

Checklist: Should You Purify Your System?

PHYSICAL MANIFESTATIONS	Yes	No
Do you suffer frequently from pimples, blackheads, boils, or other skin problems?	❑	❑
Do you often break out into a sweat for no apparent reason?	❑	❑
Do you often suffer from constipation, diarrhea, bloating, a feeling of fullness, acid indigestion, etc.?	❑	❑

Checklist: Should You Purify Your System?

PHYSICAL MANIFESTATIONS	Yes	No
Do you frequently have bad breath or strong body odor?	❏	❏
Are you overweight?	❏	❏
Do you have dents in your thighs, or cellulitis?	❏	❏
Do you often suffer from muscle cramps in the area of the shoulders and neck?	❏	❏
Do you have pain in your joints?	❏	❏
Do you get colds frequently?	❏	❏
Are you being treated by a physician for gallstones or kidney stones?	❏	❏
Do you often display signs of poor circulation such as numbness, tingling, dizziness, forgetfulness, lack of concentration, difficulty when climbing stairs?	❏	❏

NUTRITION

	Yes	No
Do you often eat without being hungry?	❏	❏
Do you prefer to eat your main meal at night?	❏	❏
Do you eat meat, sausages, or eggs almost daily?	❏	❏
Do you eat little fruit, few vegetables, and few salads?	❏	❏
Do you prefer white bread over whole-grain bread?	❏	❏
Do you frequently eat chocolate, cake, or other sweets?	❏	❏
Does it normally take you less than 10 minutes to eat soup, a main course, and dessert?	❏	❏

The more questions you mark with a "yes" in the opposite checklist, the more strongly a cure of purification is recommended for you.

Is your lifestyle good for your health? The checklist below will give you a fast and clear answer.

Checklist: Should You Purify Your System?

NUTRITION	Yes	No
Do you drink more than two cups of coffee daily?	❑	❑
Do you eat because you are bored or sad?	❑	❑
Do you always eat everything that is on your plate?	❑	❑
ENVIRONMENT		
Do you live next to a main traffic artery?	❑	❑
Do you live in an industrial region with heavy air pollution?	❑	❑
When buying food, do you seldom pay attention to ingredients or where it was grown or produced?	❑	❑
Does your job require you to work in polluted air?	❑	❑
Do you even occasionally come into contact with toxic material?	❑	❑
LIFESTYLE		
Do you smoke more than three (women) or five (men) cigarettes per day?	❑	❑
Do you drink alcohol daily?	❑	❑
Do you spend less than an hour outside daily ?	❑	❑
Do you engage in sports activities that cause you to perspire less than once or twice a month ?	❑	❑
Do you watch more than three hours of television daily?	❑	❑
Do you work primarily while sitting down?	❑	❑
Is doing nothing your favorite pastime?	❑	❑
Are you a workaholic?	❑	❑
Are athletic activities drudgery to you?	❑	❑

The Organs of Detoxification

The Body's "Sewage Treatment Plants"

Our body is not helpless against the onslaught of toxins from the outside or against its own waste products, the deposits. The body has four major "sewage treatment plants," or organs of detoxification, which rid the organism of unwanted substances. These organs are the kidneys, the lungs, the skin, and the liver (in the digestive system).

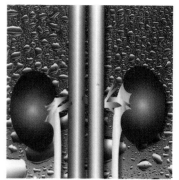

The body has four major detoxification organs, including the kidneys.

Our Reservoir of Fluids

These detoxifying organs cleanse mostly fluids. The human body consists of 60 percent water, which means that more than 50 percent of the body is made up of fluids, including blood, fluid of the connective tissue, lymph fluid, and cellular fluid; furthermore, there are about 9 liters (9½ quarts) of glandular fluid. These fluids are interconnected through various processes of exchange and form a uniform reservoir of fluids. Every disturbance—every toxin or deposit in the body—will influence this reservoir. Measures of purification or detoxification stimulating individual organs will ultimately cleanse the entire reservoir of fluids in the body. And because these fluids influence all parts of the body right down to each single cell, individual measures of detoxification will have a positive effect on the whole organism.

"What the kidneys and bladder cannot eliminate the intestines have to eliminate; what the intestines cannot eliminate the lungs have to eliminate; what the lungs cannot eliminate the skin has to eliminate, and what the skin cannot eliminate will lead to death." (old Chinese proverb)

If indigestible food residues are not eliminated, they will start to ferment in the body.

The Digestive System

In the course of the digestive process, nutrients—carbohydrates, fats, and proteins—that had been absorbed are being decomposed into their basic building blocks: sugar molecules, fatty acids, and amino acids. It is only in this changed state that the body can use the ingested nutrients for energy and for building cells.

The Absorption of Nutrients

Digestion starts in the mouth, where food is reduced to small pieces and mixed with saliva. By way of the esophagus, the chyme is brought to the stomach, where it is decomposed with the help of stomach acid; then it is transported to the small intestines. The innumerable diverticula of the small intestines absorb the decomposed nutrients and direct them to the lymph and mainly to the liver. Before the nutrients can nourish the blood's circulatory system and the rest of the body, they have to be subjected in the liver to one more transformation. Then residues of food pass through the large intestines and are eliminated after 18 to 24 hours.

Detoxification by Means of the Large Intestines

Constipation, or sluggish, or irregular, elimination can lead to the danger of slow, self-induced poisoning. Physicians in antiquity knew this, for they believed that all evil resides in the intestines.

Regular bowel movements are one of the most important processes of detoxification. Undigested residues of food, if not eliminated, will start to ferment and thus produce a series of toxins.

What Well-Functioning Intestines Can Do

Regular bowel movements not only eliminate from the organism material brought in from the outside, but also get rid of body-generated waste.

The diverticula in the mucous membrane of the intestines take in nutrients as well as pass waste products and toxins from the blood's circulatory system to the intestines. These waste products are generated primarily by cell metabolism. At any given time, only half of the body's cells are functioning fully, with one quarter dying and the other quarter growing.

When cells disintegrate, broken-down cell substances are set free, and most of them are excreted by means of the intestines.

Rejuvenation After a Few Days

Detoxification of the intestines not only produces a healthy environment within the intestines, but also can have a healing effect on all the cells of the body. Everyone can feel the positive effects of a detoxification of the intestines after a few days. Attitude, posture, breathing, joints, the skin—all will improve noticeably.

Zest for living, good posture, and glowing skin can be achieved without pills simply by detoxifying the intestines.

What Will Keep the Intestines Healthy?

➤ A wholesome diet rich in fiber
Your diet should contain fresh fruit and vegetables in season, legumes, grains, and milk products, and only small amounts of meat, fat, salt, and sweets. All ingredients should be processed as little as possible. Fiber is the indigestible matter in a vegetable diet containing cellulose, hemicellulose, lignin, and pectin. Fiber produces little energy but assures a good digestion.

> ➤ Few laxatives

Laxatives (even those derived from plants) reduce your potassium level and can injure your intestines and your heart muscles. Treat constipation instead with linseed or prunes or by drinking a glass of lukewarm water, fruit juice, or sauerkraut juice after rising in the morning.

➤ Kitchen hygiene

Bacteria like salmonella are transmitted frequently by animal products and often will produce intestinal cramps, diarrhea, and malaise. Infections of this sort need to be treated by a physician. Preventive measures: Boil eggs at least 5 minutes and don't rinse them under cold water, and when preparing fowl, thoroughly wash silverware, the cutting board, plates, and, most importantly, your hands.

➤ Regular bowel movements

Train your bowels to evacuate regularly. A regulated lifestyle with regulated food intake will help you achieve this training. In the morning and in the evening, allow yourself plenty of time to go to the bathroom, and don't suppress a bowel movement.

The Liver Barrier

Weighing up to 2 pounds, the liver is the largest gland in the body. It is situated like a large triangle on the upper-right part of your stomach. The liver is connected to the stomach by the portal vein. The liver uses the nutrients from the blood of the portal vein and filters out foreign matter and toxins by rendering them as harmless as possible.

This process is achieved with the help of chemical procedures like esterification, methylation, or the binding of toxins to amino acids. Especially toxic ammonia, produced by bacteria in the intestines during the decomposition of protein, is neutralized by the liver, which changes toxic ammonia into urea. Urea is then trans-

You probably don't have much time in the morning. But do take a few minutes for breakfast and going to the bathroom. Do it for the sake of your health.

ported by means of the blood's circulatory system to the kidneys for elimination.

Chemical Cleansing of the Liver

The liver filters about 1½ liters (or quarts) of blood in a minute. During this process, it neutralizes food additives, toxic eliminations of microorganisms, harmful substances from medicines, cholesterol, toxins produced by fermentation and putrefaction, and alcohol.

The manifold chemical tasks of the liver can be disturbed if the liver is overtaxed. Should the liver be overburdened with too much alcohol and too many medications, environmental toxins, and drugs, then the liver barrier could be crossed and the organism could be infiltrated directly, or the liver could become damaged and finally fatal cirrhosis of the liver could set in.

What Will Keep the Liver Healthy?

➤ Watching your alcohol consumption
It has been established that someone who drinks daily, over a period of 15 to 20 years, a liter of wine, half a liter of hard liquor, or two liters of beer must expect to contract cirrhosis of the liver. (A liter is equivalent to 1.057 quarts.)
➤ Hygiene
Impure water or food or stale drinks may contain extremely harmful substances for the liver like hepatitis viruses, which can cause an inflammation of the liver. Thus, you should be very careful eating and drinking when traveling in tropical regions.
➤ Proper Nutrition
People who live almost exclusively on simple carbohydrates (commercial sugar, white bread, noodles made from white flour, sweets) and, at the same time, consume almost no protein, run the risk, just like an alcoholic does, of developing a diseased liver.

The liver disposes of almost every toxic bomb—for example, toxic ammonia is turned into urea. But if the liver is constantly being overburdened, its capacity to do so declines rapidly.

➤ An overall reduced intake of toxins

Avoid all drugs and medications, and buy organic food. It often is better to drink bottled water or mineral water rather than tap water.

The Kidneys

A kidney has a length of about 12 centimeters (4½ inches) and weighs about 150 grams (5¼ ounces). From each kidney, a ureter leads to the bladder. Each kidney is connected to the blood's circulatory system by an artery carrying blood and a vein removing blood.

The Two Filtering Systems of the Kidneys

The adipose capsule of each kidney comprises 1 to 1.3 million small glomeruli that serve as blood filters. The primary urine filtered from the blood contains, besides harmful substances, useful nutrients, like sugar, amino acid, and vitamin C. This is why the primary urine is filtered through a second filtering system, the tubuli. The tubuli are so small that when added together, they have a length of about 10 kilometers (a little more than 6 miles). Here, the smallest of the blood vessels transfer nutrients still contained in the primary urine to the

Highly efficient filters, the kidneys clean all the blood of the human organism 340 to 360 times a day.

The Kidneys—Detoxification of the Organism

The most important function of the kidneys is detoxifying the organism. Along with the urine, which consists of 95 percent water, numerous harmful substances and toxins are secreted, such as urea, uric acid, excess of sodium chloride, phenol, cresol, tyrosine, minerals that can't be used by the body, and finally large amounts of environmental chemical substances taken in with our food.

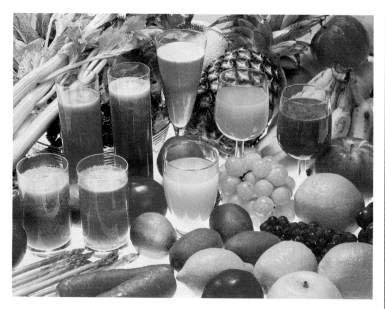

The kidneys are able to purify your body only if you drink enough liquids. You should drink 2 to 3 liters, or quarts, daily.

blood's circulatory system. By means of the ureter, the final urine filled with harmful substances flows into the bladder. This way, the kidneys, on a single day, clean all the blood in the body 340 to 360 times. During this process, about 1 to 1½ liters (or quarts) of urine are produced daily.

What Will Keep the Kidneys Healthy?

➤ Sufficient fluid
We should all drink 2 to 3 liters (or quarts) of liquid daily, even though we may not be thirsty.
➤ Warmth
The kidneys are especially sensitive to cold. Be careful when sitting on cold tile floors. After swimming, take off your wet swimsuit immediately. In winter, make sure you wear warm underwear and generally dress warmly.
➤ Normal blood pressure
If your blood pressure is too low or too high, you endanger your kidneys. Should either be the case, consult a physician.

➤ Urinating without pain

If you have problems urinating (either you are urinating too frequently or your urination is painful), you must be treated by a physician; otherwise, a chronic kidney problem could develop.

The Lungs

The lungs are our organs for breathing. With their help, we take in oxygen. After we have taken in air by way of the trachea to the bronchi, the air will travel along the fine branches of the bronchi, the bronchioles, which are spread throughout the lungs. Tiny blood vessels in the lung sacs (alveoli) take up the oxygen contained in the air and distribute it afterward throughout the organism. During this process, oxygen molecules are bound to the red blood cells and ride along. Together, the right and the left lung contain about 400 million alveoli. They not only provide the body with oxygen, but also help the body detoxify. You breathe out carbon dioxide (CO_2) brought by way of the blood. About 5 percent of the air we exhale consists of this gas.

As many as 400 million alveoli are occupied to assure the necessary oxygen supply for your body.

How You Will Start Coughing

The alveoli are passageways for several other materials. Toxins and other poisons generated by the body are flooded in by way of the blood. They are capable of making the thin walls of the alveoli permeable and can get to the outside, to the bronchiole. From there, they are transported to the top with the help of cilia at a speed of about 15 centimeters (almost 6 inches) per hour. Then by coughing or clearing your throat, they are eliminated from the breathing tract. You should never suppress a cough, and, if possible, you should spit out the secretion. This sputum not only contains toxins produced by the

Cleansing Your Body by Exhaling

Exhaling frees the body not only from used air, but also from toxins. The more forcefully you exhale when engaged in physical activity or doing breathing exercises, the more you will contribute to the inner cleansing of your body.

metabolism, but also dust or soot particles from inhaled air that could be polluted by environmental toxins.

A Tip for Those with Bronchitis

If you suffer from bronchitis (inflammation of the bronchi), you can lessen your coughing by keeping your thorax in a horizontal position. By the way, bronchitis is often not only brought on by smoking or polluted air (perhaps you live in an industrial region), but also by being overloaded with toxins.

What Will Keep Your Lungs Healthy?

➤ Don't smoke
The more you smoke, the greater the risk will be that your lungs will get damaged seriously.
➤ Increase your power of resistance
In order to protect the lungs from infections, like influenza viruses, all measures that strengthen the immune system are recommended, such as cold-water treatments, saunas, plenty of exercise in fresh air, a correct diet (with a lot of vitamins C and E), and enough sleep.
➤ Clean air
Spend as much time as you can in air free of harmful substances—for example, in fresh air up in the mountains or at the beach.
➤ Breathe correctly
Most people breathe too shallowly—that is, only in the

Are you breathing correctly? Many people breathe too shallowly. Every now and then, inhale deeply and fill your lungs with fresh air.

upper thoracic region. If you breathe correctly, not only your thorax but your stomach and your sides should move, too.

The Skin

The skin is not merely a protective covering for the body, but also an organ with diverse functions:
➤ With the nerves of our skin, we can feel the environment.
➤ The sweat glands and blood vessels of our skin regulate body temperature.
➤ The sweat and sebaceous glands along the hairline produce a protective film that prevents the growth of harmful bacteria.
➤ The skin functions as an ancillary respiratory organ, taking in a small amount (2 percent) of the necessary oxygen.
➤ The skin's ability to eliminate toxins is especially important for our metabolism.

The Skin as a Third Kidney

The skin is often called a third kidney, because by means of the sweat and sebaceous glands numerous waste products are removed from the body. The main waste products are uric acid, sodium chlorides (cooking salts), lactic acid, and acetic acid, but toxins like mercury and bromine are removed as well. Sweat, according to its composition, is undiluted urine, but sweat in cases of acute illness can contain more harmful substances than urine. Only well-functioning skin will guarantee that the body will not suffocate in waste products and toxins. The adipose tissue (connective tissues in which fat is stored) functions also as a storage for energy. In comparison to muscle and nerve tissue, the adipose tissue constitutes a less valuable tissue

A place for temporary garbage storage, the skin can safely hold waste products and toxins for a while.

26

that the body can dispense with easiest. Therefore, reducing fat always has a detoxifying effect.

What Will Keep the Skin Healthy?

Protection

➤ If you come into contact with harsh chemicals when cleaning, wear rubber gloves.

➤ Skin creams and makeup will prevent dust and dirt particles from clogging your pores. But in the evening, be sure to clean your face thoroughly.

➤ As a protection against harmful ultraviolet rays, you should always wear, in addition to a day cream, some sunscreen lotion, even when you are in the shade or on a somewhat cloudy day. If you sunbathe for an extended period of time, you must use a sun-screen lotion with a high protection factor.

➤ As a prevention against athlete's foot, wear light shoes and cotton socks, cut your toenails short, and, after washing your feet, make sure you dry the spaces between your toes well.

➤ Water treatments, plenty of sunlight and fresh air, and regular exercise also are recommended.

Skin Care

➤ Washing too frequently is harmful to your skin, as it destroys its layer of acid protection. When you wash, try to use soap free of alkali and perfume.

➤ Use mild bath oils rather than leaching bubble bath. Each time you wash your hands, moisturize them.

➤ Vitamins—especially beta carotene, which can be found in carrots, spinach, dandelion leaves, apricots, and liver—are important for your skin and your eyes.

➤ The skin needs a great deal of moisture. Walks in the rain, steam baths, moisturizing cream, and as little exposure to dry air generated by heaters as possible will keep your skin tight and healthy.

Too much washing will dry out your skin. This is why you should moisturize your hands after you wash them.

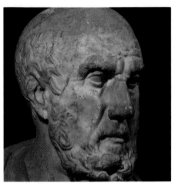

Known as the "father of medicine," Hippocrates valued the body's methods of detoxification.

The organism knows various ways of eliminating toxins. In order to detoxify, first deep-seated toxins have to be loosened.

Targeted Means of Detoxification

"All diseases are cured because of an elimination either by means of the body's orifices, the mouth, anus, bladder, or by means of the organs of elimination. The sweat glands are one of the organs that are helpful for all complaints."
— Hippocrates, Greek physician, 460–375 B.C.

The Cleansing

The interior cleansing of the body always takes place by means of the organs of elimination. With the aid of a measure of detoxification, first a specific organ of elimination, such as the liver or kidneys, will be cleansed. There are visible means of testing the effectiveness of the cleansing, including a change in bowel movements, dark strong-smelling urine, profuse perspiration, or bad breath. After the cleansing of the organ has been completed and it can function properly once more, then waste products and toxins that are found deeper inside the tissues will be dissolved and excreted.

Doses Are Important

The doses of a means of detoxification are critical in implementing a cure. If the doses are too low, then the treatment will be ineffective. If the doses are too high, then the body could be overburdened by the flood of freed toxins. Dosages cannot always be prescribed exactly, however, because every organism reacts differently.

Therefore, the dosages given in this book are only meant to serve as guidelines. You yourself must find out which dose of a means of detoxification yields the best results for you. It is best to start with small amounts and increase them gradually.

The Length of the Detoxification Process

How long you detoxify your body also is of importance. The decomposition of toxins takes place over a period of time. Light detoxification measures, as a rule, should be stretched out over several weeks.

It you undertake a strong detoxification, start with a single organ first. Then proceed, one by one, to a cleansing of the rest of the organs of elimination.

The decomposition of toxins is not possible all at once; it usually will take several weeks until impurities and toxins will have been flushed out.

Who Needs Gentle Detoxification?

The gentle forms of detoxification are especially recommended for older and weaker individuals, but also for people who are very contaminated due to faulty nutrition, heavy smoking, or misuse of drugs or alcohol.

In general, one detoxification procedure is sufficient for each organ of elimination. But if the effect of one doesn't seem strong enough, various means of detoxification can be combined.

What Are the Means of Detoxification?

There are several methods of detoxification that stimulate the organs of elimination, including the use of special medicinal herbs or foods, massage, measures to cleanse the intestines, and sweat cures.

Measures of Detoxification for the Intestines

With the aid of detoxification, the intestines are activated and cleansed. The content of the intestines consists of chyme and useless leftover material, the feces. The latter can become hardened and form a crust, which can be deposited on the walls of the intestines, if, for example, the chyme remains in the intestines too long. This "dirt" in the intestines can prevent adequate transportation of fecal matter and chyme, impair the uptake of nutrients, and affect the elimination of metabolic products.

If possible, avoid taking chemical laxatives. Generally, they are too strong and your body gets used to them quickly.

The goals of detoxifying the intestines are to repair the normal flow in the intestines and to restore the mucous membrane of the intestines. An impaired mucous membrane could cause toxins and irritating matter from food that has not been decomposed completely to enter the blood's circulatory system. But when the intestines are cleansed, products of metabolic decomposition can enter the intestines more easily and leave the body from there.

Avoid Chemical Laxatives

Chemical laxatives should be used as a purgative only in exceptional cases (total constipation or blockage) because they destroy a large amount of the intestinal flora and can lead to an infection of the mucous membrane of the intestines. If chemically based laxatives are used regularly and over a long period of time, dependency sets in which results in increased lazy bowel syndrome.

The mild natural laxatives mentioned below should lead to about two or three bowel movements a day. Increase the doses if these results do not occur. On the other hand, if you experience a greater frequency of bowel movements, or your bowel movements tend to be runny and if the intestines are being irritated, choose smaller doses or change to a different means of detoxification. You also can stop the measure you have chosen for a couple of days.

Food That Can Be Used as Laxatives

➤ Sufficient fiber (cellulose, for example) in food fills the intestines and stimulates peristalsis, the muscular movement of the intestines. Fiber can be found in fruit, vegetables, and whole-wheat products.

Fruit and Vegetable Days

➤ For a while, replace one meal a with just fruit or vegetables. Eating nothing but fruit and vegetables for a day will have a mild laxative effect as well. It is best to choose fruit and vegetables in season. Enjoy the fruit raw or as a sauce or compote (without sugar—if necessary, use artificial sweetener). Eat vegetables raw or slightly cooked, or in the form of a thick potato-vegetable soup (see sidebar).

Three Simple Food Treatments

➤ Figs and prunes
This treatment can be used for several months to stimulate digestion. Soak three figs or five prunes in a little water the evening before. Eat the fruit the next morning on an empty stomach, and drink in small gulps the water in which they had been soaking.
➤ Wheat germ
Throughout the day, eat 3 to 5 tablespoons of wheat germ mixed with yogurt, soup, or another dish. Drink at least a glass of some form of liquid per each tablespoon of wheat germ.
➤ Linseed
Add 2 to 3 tablespoons of finely broken linseed to your

Thick Potato-Vegetable Soup
Cut into cubes vegetables of your choice and 2 small potatoes with or without skin, and put into 1 liter (or quart) of cold water. Add 3 teaspoons of dried vegetable broth. Bring to a boil, and let simmer, covered, on low heat for 20 minutes. Then puree the vegetables, and season with herbs (parsley, chives, and lovage) and yeast flakes. You may want to add a tablespoon of sour cream.

TIP
People suffering from ulcers or inflammation of the large intestines should cook fruit and vegetables rather than eat them raw.

breakfast muesli, to a soup, or to vegetables. Always drink lots of liquids.

Medicinal Herbs

Most medicinal blossoms, fruit, roots, seeds, and herbs are available at health food stores and whole-foods markets. There are also stores that specialize in herbs.

Diverse Herbs

➤ Buckthorn

The black berries of buckthorn (*Rhamnus catharticus*) have a mild laxative effect. The buckthorn bush, which is about 3 meters (almost 10 feet) high, grows near hedges, at the edges of forests, and in swamps. It has branches that end in a straight thorn. The berries ripen in September or October. Only pick ripe, black berries. You can either eat 10 to 15 fresh berries on an empty stomach in the morning (chew slowly), or drink a cup of tea made from dried berries in the evening (see sidebar for preparation).

Caution!

Ingesting too many buckthorn berries could have a toxic effect. Do not take the berries for more than one to two weeks, and never take them while pregnant.

➤ Bark of the alder tree

The bark of the alder tree (*Frangula algus*) is a mild but very effective plant-based laxative. Furthermore, it stimulates the gallbladder.

The bark of the alder tree frequently is an ingredient in prepared laxative teas for the spring cure (see sidebar). You can buy the bark of the alder tree already cut and preserved for about a year or in pill form at many pharmacies and health food stores. If you buy the pills, be sure to follow the directions on the package.

You should only collect medicinal plants on your own if you have exact knowledge of their species, their preparation, and their effect.

Tea from Buckthorn Berries
Add 2 heaping teaspoons of dried buckthorn berries to ¼ liter (or quart) of cold water, bring to a boil, and strain after 2 to 3 minutes.

Tea from Alder Tree Bark
Pour cold water over 1 teaspoon of preserved alder tree bark, and let steep for 12 hours, stirring frequently. Then strain and drink before going to sleep. Do not use this tea longer than two weeks.

➤ Wild agrimony

Wild agrimony (*Anserniae herba*) tea (see sidebar) promotes the elimination of waste products and toxins by means of the intestines and kidneys, and has a soothing effect on the entire digestive system. It also soothes the reproductive organs and relaxes tense muscles, making it helpful for menstrual pain as well. Drink a cup twice or three times a day.

Incidentally, "top" is the term for the upper non-wooded part of the plant.

Tea from Wild Agrimony
Pour ¼ liter (or quart) of boiling water over 3 tea-spoons of wild agrimony. Steep for 10 minutes and strain.

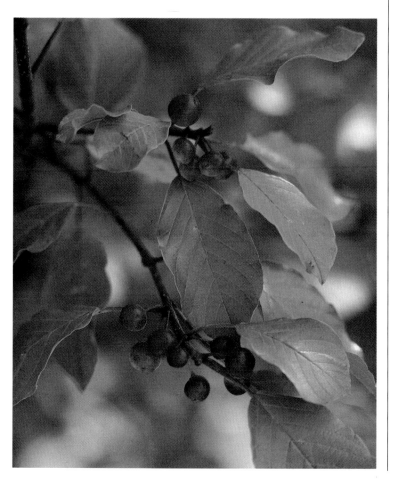

Ingesting buckthorn, wild agrimony, and the bark of the alder tree (pictured here) are highly effective means for detoxification. Teas brewed from these plants have an interesting taste.

Purgative Salts

Glauber salts (natrium sulfate) and Epsom salt (magnesium sulfate) can be obtained at pharmacies, and both have an excellent purgative effect, playing an important role in almost all fasting and detoxification protocols. With the help of these saline purgatives, the stomach and intestines are gently flushed, thereby loosening crusts on the sides of the intestines and directing them to the anus. The saline solution stimulates secretion in the liver, gallbladder, and the other digestive glands, and supports the entire digestive system in its task of detoxifying the body.

Glauber and Epsom salts are important components of almost all fasting and detoxification cures. They can be bought at your pharmacy.

Flushing Out the Intestines

With the help of an enema, water is flushed into the end of the large intestines. Thereby, the fecal matter is liquefied and crusts are loosened from the mucous membranes of the lower intestines. The water produces diarrhea defecation.

To flush out your intestines, you can use one to two enemas daily over a period of one to two weeks.

Enemas

When detoxifying or fasting, enemas are used to cleanse the intestines. This way, the large intestines will

Application of the Purgative Salts

During the detoxification cure, drink in the morning on an empty stomach a glass of water with 1 to 2 teaspoons of Epsom or Glauber salts. To improve the taste, add some lemon or some fruit juice and drink a cup of herbal tea afterward. Soon your bowels will evacuate, so stay near the bathroom.

be emptied thoroughly, and detoxified. Two methods are presented here.

Method One

This method is the simplest, and requires only an enema bag with a plastic hose or applicator, which you can buy at a drugstore.

➤ Fill the enema bag with water at body temperature. If you prefer, you can add some infusion of chamomile to prevent infections.

➤ Grease the end of the plastic hose or the applicator with Vaseline or vegetable oil, and introduce it into the anus.

➤ While standing, pump the water into the intestines.

➤ Don't hold the water back, but go to the toilet right away.

➤ Repeat this procedure several times until the appearance of your stool becomes clearer and clearer.

Method Two

For this method, you will need an irrigator with a water bag, a rubber hose, and an extension with a faucet. If you can't find this at a drugstore, a medical supply store will have it.

➤ Fill the water bag with of water at body temperature. Hang up the enema bag in an elevated position—for example, on a towel rack or the doorknob.

➤ Grease the extension part with Vaseline or vegetable oil.

➤ Go down to the floor on all fours.

➤ Introduce the extension with the faucet closed into your anus.

➤ Open the faucet, and slowly let the water flow in.

➤ Try to hold back the water (for about 5 to 10 minutes) so that the stool can liquefy and residues can be loosened; then go to the toilet.

The enema consists of a bag and a plastic hose or an applicator attached to it.

Enemas for cleansing the intestines are not for everyone. Here, you can find out how to do it.

Detoxification Measures for the Liver and Gallbladder

If the Liver Gives Out

If the metabolism of your liver does not function well, you might experience, especially after a heavy meal, malaise, a feeling of satiety, flatulence, a headache, dizziness, and fatigue, and have a white-coated tongue.

Natural Ways to Detoxify

What relieves your intestines will also ease the burden on your liver. Therefore, when emptying out your intestines, you will help yourself twice.

Natural detoxification measures that will stimulate the work of the liver and elicit the output of bile into the alimentary tract are cures with certain fruits and vegetables or medicinal plants and heat treatments. An indication that these means of detoxification are working could be an acceleration in the passing of stools. It is important to note that if diarrhea occurs, then the cleansing method is too strong.

From One Purification to the Next

After the liver has been purified, it can once more perform its original tasks: eliminating toxic substances taken in with food and filtering metabolic waste from the blood.

It should be mentioned that each purification of the intestines also will affect the liver and gallbladder (in which bile from the liver is stored), because the liver is connected indirectly to the intestines by means of the portal vein. What eases the burden of the intestines also will relieve the liver. And what eases the burden of the liver also will help your entire organism to purify and detoxify.

Food That Will Stimulate the Liver and Gallbladder

The following fruits and vegetables will activate the purification work of the liver and the excretion of bile (important for the reduction of fat): foremost are plums, but also pineapple, apples, strawberries, black currants, cherries, gooseberries, grapes, and citrus fruit, as well as eggplant, avocados, potatoes, carrots, cabbage, celery, and asparagus.

An Artichoke Cure

➤ This treatment stimulates in the liver the production of bile and incites the gallbladder to eliminate bile, acts as a diuretic, and lowers cholesterol.

For several weeks, drink three times a day 2 teaspoons of artichoke juice (available at health food stores), or a tea made from the leaves of artichokes (see sidebar). You also should eat artichoke hearts, and the inner leaves, as a vegetable as frequently as possible.

Dandelion Salad—Delicious and Healthful

➤ The tender leaves of dandelion, gathered in April and May and then prepared as a salad, taste delicious, stimulate the liver, gallbladder, and kidneys, and provide for a stronger blood flow within the connective tissue.

Dandelion juice is especially well suited for a detoxification cure of four to six weeks. It can prevent the new formation or enlargement of gallstones in individuals with such a tendency. Twice a day, drink a tablespoon of dandelion juice (available at health food stores), or a cup of dandelion tea (see sidebar) in small gulps.

TIP
Before every heavy meal, enjoy, as an aperitif, a small glass of dandelion juice.

Tea from Artichoke Leaves
Pour boiling water over less than a tablespoon of artichoke leaves, let steep for 10 minutes, and strain. Drink three times a day before meals.

Dandelion Tea
Pour ¼ liter (or quart) of cold water over 2 teaspoons of dandelion plant and root, heat, and let boil for 1 minute; then steep for 10 minutes. (Caution! The stems of fresh dandelion, when eaten in large quantities, are supposedly unhealthy.)

Radish Juice

➤ The juice of black radishes (see procedure in sidebar) stimulates the production of bile, prevents gallbladder infections and formation of gallstones, and protects the liver.
➤ Radish juice can be bought in some health food stores, or you can make it yourself with a food processor or a juicer.
➤ You can buy radishes at the grocery store or grow them yourself in your garden.

Olive Oil and Tea

➤ Olives, olive oil, as well as the leaves of the olive tree, are well suited for purification of the liver and gallbladder; furthermore, the leaves are effective in treating high blood pressure. (See the sidebar for how to make tea from olive leaves).
➤ Use only cold-pressed extra virgin olive oil.
➤ For two weeks, take every morning 2 tablespoons of olive oil with a few drops of lemon on an empty stomach.
➤ Repeat the treatment several times a year. It stimulates the production of bile and helps digestion.
➤ This cure with olive oil, however, is not suited for people who have problems with their digestion.

Yarrow

➤ Because of its tannic acid and bitter principle and its high content of potassium as well as ethereal oils, yarrow (*Millefolii herba*) not only supports the detoxification process of the liver but also soothes varicose veins and hemorrhoids.
➤ A tea made from yarrow (see sidebar) is therefore one of the most effective measures you can take for the purification of the blood and other body fluids and for a general detoxification.

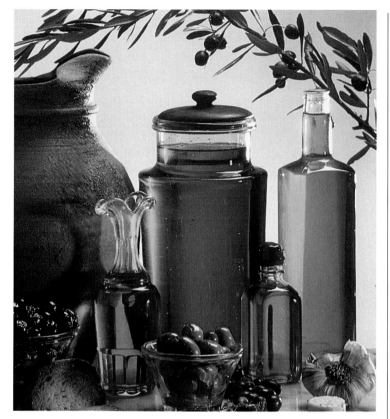

Cold-pressed olive oil is not merely delicious, but also an excellent medicine. A treatment with olive oil purifies the body naturally.

Medicinal Plants: Centaury and Vermouth

You can either buy medicinal plants already prepared at health food stores or pick the blooming plants yourself in meadows from July to September. Once you have collected them, hang the plants up to dry and remove their wooded stems.

➤ The bitter principle of centaury (*Erythraea centaurium*) helps with problems of the liver and gallbladder and stimulates the digestive process. Centaury also has been shown to be useful for cleansing the blood and in cases of anemia. It can be bought in health food stores. The plant is rela-

Centaury Tea
Pour ¼ liter (or quart) of cold water over 2 teaspoons of the chopped plant, let steep for 6 to 8 hours, and then strain and reheat. Before meals, drink 1 cup of the unsweetened tea.

Vermouth Tea
Pour ¼ liter (or quart) of
boiling water over 1 to 2 tea-
spoons of cut vermouth, steep
for 10 minutes, and strain.
Drink 1 to 2 unsweetened
cups daily.

TIP
Before a heavy meal, enjoy a
small glass of vermouth wine
as an aperitif.

Hildegard von Bingen left numerous naturopathic recipes. Only gradually are people starting to value again the benefits of natural healing methods.

tively rare, so it is not easy to pick yourself. (To prepare tea from the centaury plant, see the sidebar on page 39.)

➤ The vermouth plant (*Absinthii herba*), thanks to its ethereal oils, is an excellent means for cleansing the blood, stimulating digestion, and alleviating stomach and gallbladder trouble.

A small glass of vermouth taken every three days on an empty stomach will cleanse all your inner organs. A small amount of vermouth also will support the reduction of fat during the digestive process. (To prepare vermouth tea, see the sidebar.)

Recipe for Vermouth Wine

Ingredients: 1 liter (or quart) of wine, about 10 tablespoons of honey, and about 3 tablespoons of vermouth juice (from the health food store).

Preparation: Pour the wine into a pot, and bring it slowly to a boil. Stir in the honey. Take the wine off the stove, and add enough vermouth juice so that the taste of the vermouth juice will surpass the taste of the honey and the wine, which means a somewhat bitter vermouth taste should dominate. Pour into sterilized bottles and seal well. Store the vermouth wine in the refrigerator.

Hildegard's Four-Point Method of Healing

➤ Diet (correct nutrition, as well as way of life)

➤ Diverse healing and detoxification measures (from flora, fauna, metals, and precious stones)

➤ Means of elimination (for example, the nearly forgotten bloodletting and leeching)

➤ Fasting (primarily for the purpose of remembering God)

Hildegard von Bingen: Her Life and Work

The holy Hildegard von Bingen was born 1098 in Germany, in Bermersheim near Mainz. Because she was the tenth child, she was destined, according to the customs of the time, to enter a monastery. At the age of eight, Hildegard entered a Benedictine monastery, where she remained until the end of her life. In 1136 she was elected abbess. In 1147 she founded her own monastery in Rupertsberg near Bingen on the Rhine. Since childhood, Hildegard maintained that she was having divine visions. In one such vision, she was instructed to write down her divine inspirations. Three large manuscripts thus ensued: *Know the Ways (Scivias)*, *The Book of Life Merits (Liber Vitae Meritorum)*, and *The Book of Divine Works (Liber Divinorum Operum)*.

Hildegard von Bingen also was a naturopath. She alleviated the suffering of many people, and even advised crowned heads, such as Emperor Frederick I. Above all, Hildegard gathered old and well-known folk-medicine remedies and natural methods for treating illness.

Even though today not all of Hildegard's methods of treatment are of medical importance (for example, bloodletting), we nevertheless are indebted to her for the knowledge of the purifying and detoxifying properties of many plants that otherwise probably would have been forgotten. In her time, Hildegard maintained that fasting is one of the best natural methods of staying healthy, a view held by many today. The day of the holy Hildegard is September 17, the day of her death.

Four Healing Herbs

➤ The needle-shaped leaves of rosemary (*Rosmarinus officinalis*), a typical plant of the Mediterranean, are used

Rosemary, wild chicory, and peppermint contain tannic acid and bitter principle, which support the bile production of the liver.

Tea from Rosemary Leaves
Pour ¼ liter (or quart) of cold water over 1 to 2 teaspoons of rosemary leaves (bought at a health food store or grown yourself in flowerpots), bring to a boil, let steep for 5 to 10 minutes, and strain.

Wild Chicory Tea
Pour ¼ liter (or quart) of water over 1 to 2 table-spoons of the dried root or plant (or both), and bring to a boil. Let boil for about 3 minutes and steep for about 3 minutes; then strain. Drink a cup of this tea three times a day.

Peppermint Tea
Pour ¼ liter (or quart) of boiling water over 1 tea-spoon of peppermint leaves, steep for 10 minutes, and strain. Drink a cup of the unsweetened tea three times daily.

Goldenrod Tea
Pour ¼ liter (or quart) of cold water over 2 tea-spoons of goldenrod, bring to a boil, and boil for 2 min-utes; then steep for 10 min-utes, and strain. Drink 3 cups daily during a blood-purification cure.

for stomach and intestinal problems as well as for kidney, gallbladder, and liver trouble.

Drink mornings and afternoons 2 teaspoons of rosemary juice (available at the health food store), or a cup of rose-mary tea (see sidebar on page 41). Be sure not to use rose-mary tea in the evening, because it has a stimulating effect.

➤ Wild chicory (*Cichorium intybus*) contains tannic acid and bitter principle, which stimulate the liver and pro-duce bile. For purification of the blood and to alleviate metabolic disturbances, tea made from the plant or its roots is used (see sidebar). The blooming plant should be cut in July, and the root dug up in September or October. Both have to be dried.

➤ The tannic acid and bitter principle contained in the leaves of peppermint (*Mentha piperita*) support the dis-charge and production of bile in the liver. (To prepare peppermint tea, see the sidebar.)

➤ Goldenrod (*Solidago virgaurea*) is an excellent herb for ridding the body of excess water, for stimulating the metabolism in cases of kidney and bladder infections, and for purifying the gallbladder and liver. Many teas for the purification of the blood contain goldenrod. Approx-imately 1 meter (40 inches) high, the plant grows usually at the edges of forests and in meadows.

Heat Treatment

It has been proven that warmth introduced from the outside has a positive effect on the liver when the tem-perature is at about 40°C (or 104°F), or higher than normal body temperature. The warmth accelerates the flow of blood in the capillaries of the liver, which in turn speeds up the supply of nutrients to the liver cells and the cleansing of waste products. The procedure is as follows:

➤ Fill a hot-water bottle made of rubber, and put it against the upper-right side of your abdomen.
➤ Cover the bottle with a dry towel, and rest for a while. The best time to do this is after meals—for example, during an afternoon nap.

Purification Measures for the Kidneys

In the kidneys, numerous waste products (urea, uric acid, mineral salts, intestinal putrefaction products, pigments, chemical and synthetic products) are filtered from the blood and then excreted by means of the urine. If the amount of toxins in the blood is so large that it will overwhelm the capacity of the kidneys, the kidney filters will become clogged and waste products will remain in the blood.

Colorless or almost colorless urine indicates that only a few toxins are being eliminated. However, this is not true for people who drink a great deal of liquids.

Many people suffer from kidney diseases. Therefore, use prevention measures to support the kidneys in their work.

Natural Diuretics

Purification measures for the kidneys should stimulate filtration and elimination of waste products, which is why they need to have a diuretic effect. After taking such a diuretic, you will pass more urine than normally. The urine also will be darker and smell stronger—a sign that more waste products are being flushed out. Here, only natural diuretics will be introduced that you can use without side effects over an extended period of time.

More than 3,000 years ago, the healing properties of asparagus were discovered. Do you know a medicine that tastes better?

CAUTION!
If you suffer from an acute infection of the liver, you must not eat asparagus.

ONION JUICE
Finely cut 2 onions, and steep in ¼ liter (or quart) of cold water overnight. Strain in the morning and drink.

Foods That Stimulate the Production of Urine

A diuretic effect is produced by the following foods:
➤ White cabbage
People who consume 300 grams (10½ ounces) of raw, shredded cabbage daily over a period of one to two weeks will notice a stronger urine production. Cabbage juice, made in a juicer yourself or bought at the health food store, has the same diuretic effect. Cooked cabbage, however, doesn't produce this result.
➤ Cabbage juice is also beneficial in cases of ulcers, as medical tests have shown. But you will have to drink about 1 liter (or quart) of cabbage juice after each meal over a period of several weeks.

Asparagus and Fennel—Delicacies That Are Good for You

➤ Asparagus
This delicious vegetable cleanses the blood, promotes excretion of urine, stimulates the cell activities of the kidneys, and acts as a mild laxative. As far back as 3,000 years ago, people ate asparagus for medicinal purposes.
➤ Fennel
The fruit of fennel increases appetite and acts as a diuretic. Fennel is an ingredient in numerous tea mixtures for spring cures and is also used in cases of flatulence.
   To prepare fennel tea, cut some fennel fruit into slices and dry them in the open air. Pour ¼ liter (or quart) of water over 2 tablespoons of dried fennel. Boil for 5 minutes, steep for another 5 minutes, and then strain. Drink 1 cup three times daily unsweetened.

Onion Juice for the Prevention of Colds

➤ Onions

Fresh onions are a diuretic, stimulate digestion, increase appetite, produce bile, strengthen the heart, and prevent infections and colds. You should use them in as many dishes as possible. Onion juice can be bought, and 2 to 3 teaspoons daily are recommended dosages. (To prepare onion juice, see the sidebar on page 44.)

Healing Plants for the Kidneys

➤ Birch Leaves

Tea from birch (*Betula pendula*) leaves is a mild diuretic that does not irritate the kidneys. In addition to eliminating water in the body, the tea lowers high uric-acid levels. (To prepare the tea, see the sidebar.) You also may enjoy fresh birch leaves in salads.

➤ Lime blossoms

Tea from lime (*Tiliae flos*) blossoms is a diuretic and sudorific, which means that toxins will be flushed out my means of the skin as well as the kidneys. It is known as a diaphoretic (having the power to increase sweating) tea for prevention, but it also is used throughout a feverish cold. (See sidebar.)

➤ Nettle

The leaves of the two nettles that grow in Central Europe—*Urtica dioica* and *Urtica urens*—are diuretic, increase blood formation, and strengthen the entire metabolism.

Nettle tea (see sidebar) is especially good for flushing out uric acid and rheumatic toxins. Men who suffer from prostate problems drink it, too.

Gather the leaves from May to August, and dry them in the open air. If you want to make juice, use the

---

Tea from Birch Leaves
Collect birch leaves in May and June and dry them, or buy them at a health food store. Pour ¼ liter (or quart) of boiling water over 2 heaping teaspoons of dried birch leaves, steep for 10 minutes, and then strain. Drink 1 cup daily during a diaphoretic cure.

Lime-Blossom Tea
Pour ¼ liter (or quart) of boiling water over 2 to 3 teaspoons of lime blossoms, steep for 10 minutes, and then strain. Drink 1 cup two to three times daily with honey.

Tea from Nettle Leaves
Pour ¼ liter (or quart) of boiling water over 1 to 2 tablespoons of nettle leaves (gathered from June to August and air-dried); let boil for 5 minutes and steep for 5 minutes. For four weeks, drink 1 cup slowly mornings and evenings.

Fresh cherries are delicious. But only a few people know that you also can use their stems to brew a diuretic tea.

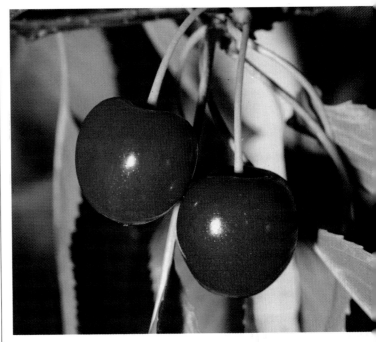

Tea from Rest Harrow
Pour ¼ liter (or quart) of boiling water over 1 to 2 tablespoons of cut-up roots, let steep for 15 minutes, and strain. Drink 2 cups daily.

Tea from Cherry Stems
Pour 1 liter (or quart) of boiling water over a handful of stems, let boil for 10 minutes, and strain. (Very dry stems should be soaked in cold water for 12 hours and then cooked in the water.) Drink ¼ liter (or quart) of the tea daily.

whole plant. You can prepare an especially delicious and healthy salad with the tender young leaves.

Nettle juice can be bought, or you can prepare it yourself. When the plant is in bloom, cut it down, and then soak it for 12 hours in a little water. Put it into the juicer. Take 2 teaspoons three times a day.

➤ Rest harrow

The root of rest harrow (*Ononis spinosa*) is effective for water retention in the body and has a positive influence on the bladder and kidney stones. In antiquity, this natural medicine was already prescribed. You can buy rest harrow in pharmacies and health food stores. (To make tea from rest harrow, see the sidebar.)

➤ Cherries

If you eat cherries, save the stems. Tea brewed from cherry stems (see sidebar) is a diuretic.

MORE MEDICINAL TEAS FOR THE KIDNEYS ■

➤ Juniper berries

A cure with dried juniper berries (*Juniperus communis*) is diuretic, cleanses the blood, and has proven to be effective for rheumatism. The dried berries can be bought at health food stores or at stores that carry herbs and spices. (See sidebar for tea preparation.)

According to a cure formulated by Sebastian Kneipp, a pastor known for various water treatments, you chew well and then swallow one berry three times on the first day of the treatment. Then you increase the amount of berries every day by one berry until you get to 20 berries. Thereafter, you decrease the amount of berries until you are eating again three berries daily. Do not use this treatment more than twice or three times a year.

Caution! If you have an acute kidney infection, you must not use juniper berries in any form. External use (bath, oil) also should be avoided.

➤ Currants

The leaves of black currants are collected in June and then air-dried. The tea prepared with the dried leaves (see sidebar) is a diuretic and also soothes the pain of rheumatism and gout. This is why the berries are sometimes called gout berries.

➤ Horsetail

The horsetail plant (*Equisetum arvese*) is a light diuretic and an ingredient in many teas for the kidneys and bladder. Because some horsetail varieties are toxic, only people who know the plant should collect it. Horsetail can be bought at health food stores. (For a tea preparation, see the sidebar.)

A bath with horsetail is recommended in cases of poor blood circulation or metabolic diseases. Pour 1 liter (or quart) of water over 100 grams (3½ ounces) of the plant, and let sit for an hour; then pour the suds into the bathwater.

Tea from Juniper Berries
Pour ¼ liter (or quart) of boiling water over 1 heaping teaspoon of dried juniper berries, steep for 10 minutes, and strain. Drink 1 cup twice daily.

Tea from Currant Leaves
Pour ¼ liter (or quart) of cold water over 2 teaspoons of the leaves, and slowly bring to a boil; then strain immediately. Drink 1 cup three times a day.

Tea from Horsetail
Pour ¼ liter (or quart) of cold water over 2 teaspoons of the cut plant, and steep for 12 hours. Then strain and heat. If you are in a hurry, pour boiling water over the plant and let it steep for 15 minutes. Drink 1 cup three times a day.

Beverages That Should Be Avoided for Quenching Thirst	
➤ Soft drinks, lemonade, and fruit nectars loaded with sugar	➤ Alcoholic beverages ➤ Coffee and black tea ➤ Milk

Drink, Drink, and Drink Again

Drinking large quantities is the best way to relieve your kidneys. Most suited are fruit and herbal teas or mineral water.

The more you drink, the more effective detoxification by means of the kidneys will be. Always drink more than your thirst requires (at least 2 to 3 liters, or quarts, a day). In order to support your body in its detoxification effort, you should drastically increase your intake of fluids. This way, you will flush your organism clean. A special drinking cure is best suited for this purpose.

What Is a Drinking Cure?

Occasionally, conduct a drinking cure, by which you will drink 3 to 4 liters (more than 3 to 4 quarts) of liquid a day. Best suited are the following:
➤ Noncarbonated mineral water
➤ Herbal and fruit teas with a little honey or lemon
➤ Thinned fruit juices without sugar
    This is the best purification measure you can undertake for your kidneys.

Avoiding Meat

The kidneys are almost solely responsible for the elimination of nitrogenous waste products from uric-acid producing (purine-containing) foods, which are mainl meat. Avoiding meat (especially organ meat) for a while or even avoiding all solid food, is highly beneficial for the kidneys.

Detoxifying the Lungs

By means of the lungs, mostly gaseous waste products and mucous impurities but also tiny dust particles (house dust, air pollution, pollen) are eliminated. The measures of detoxification for the lungs support the normal cleansing mechanisms of the lungs, such as clearing your throat, coughing, or the elimination of secretions by way of the nose.

Exercise

Inhaling and exhaling deeply—for example, when engaged in sports activities—will loosen impurities in the breathing passages. The best means of detoxification for the lungs is to increase the depth of your breathing at least once a day until you get almost out of breath. This will increase the oxygen content in your blood and other body fluids, lead to an excretion of hormones and thus elevate your mood, and stimulate blood circulation and digestion.

You will pump more oxygen into your body if you move your upper torso and your arms, which means that playing tennis or digging in your garden strenu-

Run until you are out of breath, then walk, then run again, then walk, and so on. Thus, not only will you detoxify your lungs, but you also will become fit and healthy.

How to Detoxify Your Lungs

Jogging, fast bicycling, playing tennis, and swimming, but also going up and down stairs quickly, will loosen the mucus that has accumulated in your lungs.

ously is better for detoxifying your lungs than jogging or running. But running is beneficial, too. Run for a few minutes, and as soon as you get out of breath, change to fast-paced walking. Then run again. Every day increase the time that you run.

Breathing Exercises

➤ Yoga

The more used air leaves the lungs when exhaling, the more toxins will leave the lungs and make room for fresh air when inhaling. In yoga breathing techniques, a great deal of emphasis is placed on exhaling, and inhaling will follow quite spontaneously and be short.

➤ Singing

Singing is an excellent breathing exercise because it supports exhaling. The increased expulsion of carbon dioxide is one of the reasons singers rarely ever suffer from depression.

➤ A Breathing Technique

Do this breathing technique as frequently as possible. Sit up straight in a chair and relax. Exhale as long as you can (count along in your mind), and then inhale automatically. Feel how your stomach rises and falls. Always inhale through your nose. In order to support exhaling, you also can exhale while making a "fff" sound or a slight whistling noise.

➤ The Lion Exercise

The lion exercise is a cleansing breathing exercise derived from yoga. It got its name because while doing it, you will resemble a yawning lion. The exercise has proven to be an excellent prevention against tonsillitis and a sore throat, and also is helpful in their beginning stages. If you do this exercise three times a day, you

Do you like to sing? Great. Your lungs will be happy, because singing supports the cleansing of the lungs.

will be fairly well protected against illness. At the same time, you will be cleansing your bronchi well.

You must always do this exercise outdoors in fresh air. Here is how it is performed:

➤ Stand or sit up straight.

➤ Exhale vigorously and for a long duration in the following manner.

➤ Stretch your head and neck forward (your back has to remain straight); then do the following.

➤ Open your mouth as wide as possible.

➤ Stick out your tongue as far as you can. If you feel embarrassed about being seen, try it while taking a solitary walk.

➤ Wait until you have exhaled completely and put your tongue back in your mouth; then inhale through your nose and do the following.

➤ Roll up your tongue, and press it firmly to the back of your palate.

➤ At the same time, push your chin downward as far as possible.

➤ Exhale and repeat the exercise several times. When doing the lion exercise, make sure you don't stretch your maxillary muscles too much!

Five Healing Plants for the Lungs

For detoxifying your lungs, nature offers five plants in particular: eucalyptus, plantain, coltsfoot, thyme, and dwarf pine.

➤ Eucalyptus

Inhaling eucalyptus (*Eucalyptus globulus*) tea prevents the formation of mucus in the bronchi, produces phlegm, soothes coughing, and disinfects and calms irritated and infected mucous membranes. (See sidebar for tea preparation.)

Lions—kings of the jungle. Yawn like a true lion. This lion exercise is funny and good for your lungs.

Eucalyptus Tea
Pour ¼ liter (or quart) of boiling water over 3 teaspoons of eucalyptus leaves. Steep for 15 minutes and strain. Drink 1 cup three times a day.

How to Inhale Tea Correctly

➤ Prepare ¼ liter (or quart) of medicinal plant tea, and pour it, while very hot, into a large cup or a plate.

➤ Bend your face over the vessel so that you can inhale the healing steam through your nose.

➤ Cover your head and the vessel with a towel.

➤ Inhale as long as the herbal tea is steaming.

➤ As an alternative, you can add 10 to 15 drops of an ethereal oil to boiling water. Then inhale as above. For in-between times, drip a few drops of an ethereal oil on your hand and inhale deeply.

Plantain Tea
Pour ¼ liter (or quart) of boiling water over 2 teaspoons of plantain leaves, and steep for 15 minutes. Drink 3 cups daily sweetened with honey, or inhale (without honey).

➤ Plantain

Plantain (*Plantago lanceo*), which grows in Europe in meadows, fields, and the edges of paths, is an excellent cough medicine and purifies the breathing passages. In addition, the juice pressed from fresh leaves cleanses the blood. Take 3 teaspoons a day of the juice, available at health food stores. (To prepare tea made from plantain leaves, see the sidebar.)

➤ Coltsfoot

Coltsfoot Tea
Pour ¼ liter (or quart) of boiling water over 3 teaspoons of coltsfoot, steep for 10 minutes, and strain. Drink 1 cup perhaps sweetened with honey three times a day, or inhale (without honey), but for no longer than three weeks.

Tea made from coltsfoot (*Tussilago farfara*) leaves (see sidebar) liquefies mucus in the bronchi and soothes coughing. Take 2 tablespoons daily of the juice. Coltsfoot can be found at the edges of rocky paths, in refuse dumps and in poor, rocky soil. If you pick the plant yourself, make sure it is not growing too close to streets with heavy traffic, because then the plant will have been polluted undoubtedly by car exhaust.

Not merely the leaves but the flowers as well can be used for tea. Collect the flowers, dry them, and pour hot water over them. If you do collect coltsfoot

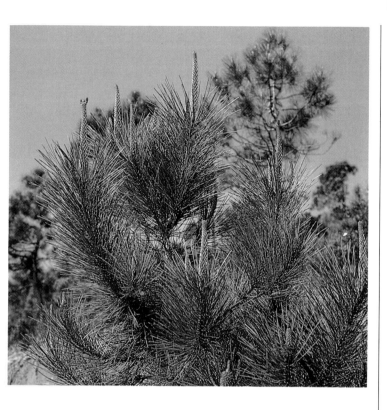

Oil of the dwarf pine is well suited for inhalation. This way, it will cleanse your lungs naturally.

plants, why not put a few in flowerpots on the windowsill?

➤ Thyme

Dried thyme *(Thymus vulgaris)*, either drunk as tea or inhaled, soothes cramps and coughs, loosens mucus, and disinfects. (To make tea from thyme, see the sidebar.)

➤ Dwarf pine

The oil from the protected dwarf pine *(Pinus montana)* is extracted from its needles. Inhalation with 10 to 15 drops of the etherial oil in ¼ liter (or quart) of water will loosen the mucus in the bronchi.

Pine needle oil can be obtained in different-sized bottles at health food stores.

Tea Made from Thyme
Pour ¼ liter (or quart) of cold water over 1 to 2 teaspoons of the plant, bring to a boil, and strain. Drink 1 cup sweetened with honey three times a day, or inhale (without honey).

How to Purify Your Skin

By means of the sebaceous glands and the pores of the skin, soluble waste products, including urine, uric acid, and salt, leave the body. And by means of the sweat glands at the end of hair roots, mainly residues from medications and products of intestinal fermentation are excreted.

The skin is the largest organ of the body. With a targeted purification of the skin, you will experience a much greater sense of well-being.

How Much Do We Perspire Daily?

Perspiration at normal body temperature amounts to ¼ to 1 liter (or quart) daily. If you have a fever, it may be 2 liters or more. In hot weather and with hard physical labor, perspiration is especially high. Most measures for the purification of the skin produce perspiration and thus an increased elimination of toxins. This is why, during intensive cures of purification (fasting), sometimes skin problems like inflammation of the sebaceous glands occur, although they soon will disappear. In addition, you should know that highly odorous perspiration is a sign of intensive elimination of waste products.

The Blood Circulation of the Skin

The skin is equipped with a widespread network of fine blood vessels, the capillaries. Under the influence of heat, the capillaries expand and become filled with blood. On the other hand, if it is cold, the capillaries will shrink and blood will be pressed to the inside of the body.

This mechanism is the foundation of all cold- and warm-water treatments, which will produce stronger blood circulation and thus an increased elimination of toxins via the skin. Treatments like dry brushing of the

Dry-Brushing Technique

➤ Starting with your right foot, brush your entire body with a dry luffa glove in circular motions always in the direction toward the heart. Brush for 2 to 3 minutes until your skin turns slightly red. Afterward, rub your body with a good skin oil.

➤ This brush massage also can be done in water while taking a bath. Finish off your bath by taking a cold shower, and then rest. When you do this, a wonderful feeling of well-being will set in. Your body will get warm, and you will feel refreshed and rejuvenated.

skin, sunbathing, and alternating hot and cold showers will clearly improve the capacity of the capillaries.

Dry Brushing

Massaging your skin by brushing it daily with a luffa glove has many benefits: not only will it stimulate the metabolism and the ability of your skin to eliminate toxins, but it will energize the involuntary nervous system and increase the flow of blood and the loosening of dead skin cells. You also can use a brush instead of a luffa glove.

Massaging with a brush or luffa glove is so simple that you can do it while taking a bath.

Sweat to Purify Your Skin

In order to increase perspiration, you can overdress when doing gymnastics, running, or digging in your garden. But make sure you are wearing clothing made from natural material (doubling up on cotton sweatshirts works well). Afterwards, take a warm shower and finish it off with a cold gush. Cold water will close your pores and strengthen your resistance.

Physical Activity

Any type of sport or physical activity produces perspiration and thus detoxification via the skin.

Inducing Perspiration

"A sweat bath is good and useful for a person who is overweight because it will limit and diminish the fluids that are superfluous."—Hildegard von Bingen, abbess and healer, 1098–1179

Steam baths and saunas are regarded highly in many countries as a way to detoxify the body and strengthen its resistance. Native Americans, for example, formerly went regularly to sweat lodges for therapeutic and ritual sweating.

The Purifying Sauna

The hot air in the sauna (60 to 90° C, or 140 to 194°F) enlarges the blood vessels and blood flows to the surface. By way of the wide-open pores, perspiration laden with toxins flows out. During the following cold shower, pores close again, the blood vessels contract, and the blood is pressed back to deeper layers. Besides having a diaphoretic (power to increase sweating) effect, during this process vascular muscles also are trained. At a single visit to the sauna, about 200 milliliters (about 6½ ounces) of sweat are secreted and, along with it, many toxins and water that has collected in the tissue (or edema). The lost fluids then will be replaced by fat tissue, which is rich in water.

The sauna has additional benefits, as it:

➤ Improves the blood circulation throughout the entire body

➤ Levels out blood pressure that is either too high or too low

> For a long time, the Finnish people have been aware of how the sauna refreshes both the body and soul. You will like the effects of the sauna, and if there are two of you, you will like them even more.

➤ Strengthens the body's defense mechanisms against infections
➤ Moistens the breathing passages and increases the elimination of mucus (important for prevention)
➤ Relaxes muscles
➤ Beautifies, rejuvenates, and moisturizes the skin
➤ Has a positive effect on the involuntary nervous system and the hormonal system
➤ Supports reduction of body weight
➤ Relaxes and fosters peace of mind

Hot and Cold Body Compresses

A milder form of sauna for in-between times is hot and cold body compresses.

Method One

➤ Dip a bath towel into hot water, wring it out, and wrap it around your body.
➤ Now wrap a dry towel and a blanket around the wet towel.
➤ Thus wrapped, go to bed and cover yourself with another blanket.
➤ Stay in bed until you start to perspire heavily.
➤ Because many toxins are excreted by means of the skin, take a warm shower afterward and finish with a cold gush of water.

Method Two

The body compress by Prießnitz has proven to be an excellent remedy in cases of insomnia and fever.
➤ First warm up by taking a sunbath or a hot bath.
➤ Dip a large bath towel in cold water, and wrap it around you.
➤ Wrap a blanket around the towel and, thus wrapped, go to bed and cover yourself with another blanket.

Sweating is one of the most important methods for cleansing the skin. By using hot and cold body compresses, you are supporting your skin in its cleansing task.

➤ Soon you will become warm. This method is best used in the evening, because in no time you will get very sleepy.

Bath with Rising Temperatures

"Bathing in hot springs brings health to human beings, because warmth will consume their bad fluids.—Abbess Hildegard von Bingen

Bathing with rising temperatures leads to a gradual warming of the body, until you will finally break out into a sweat. This is the process:

➤ Lie in a bathtub filled with water at a temperature of about 37°C (or about 98.6°F).

➤ Slowly let very hot water flow in until it becomes so hot that you can barely stand it (between 37 and 42°C, or 98.6 and 107.6°F, depending on what you are used to).

➤ Stay in the bathtub for a quarter of an hour. You can gradually increase the duration of the bath each time from 5 to 15 minutes.

➤ If you feel like it, drink a perspiration-producing tea from elderberry flowers beforehand.

➤ For a cooling effect, put a cold washcloth on your forehead.

➤ Get up carefully, and take a warm shower to remove toxins eliminated with the perspiration. Finish with a cool-to-cold shower.

➤ Rest afterwards, well covered, for at least a quarter of an hour.

It is best to take this bath every two days during a

Taking a bath with rising temperatures is an excellent way to purify your skin. Here, you will find out how to do it.

TIP
A bath with rising temperatures also can be performed as a foot, leg, or sitz bath.

Important!
If you have problems with your heart or your circulatory system, it is not advisable to take a bath with rising temperatures.

CAUTION	
If you don't feel well (weakness, dizziness, feeling of oppression),	interrupt the bath immediately and refresh your body with cool water.

cure of purification because, aside from relaxation, it also promotes sleep.

Water Treatment with Kneipp's Gushes

The gushes can be warm, cold, or alternating between warm and cold, but the final gush should be cold. The stream of water has to be uniform, and you shouldn't use a shower head.

If you use alternating cold and warm gushes, direct the warm stream of water to a part of your body until it feels warm and relaxed; afterward, use a stream of cold water for the same place for 15 seconds to a minute. Start the Kneipp's gushes always at a place farthest away from the heart. Be sure the bathroom where you perform the treatment is well heated. After the procedure, rub yourself dry with a towel until your skin turns slightly red and your body is warm. You also can just brush off the wetness with your hands, and then go to bed.

Showers and Gushes

➤ Alternating hot and cold showers
These cleanse the blood, detoxify, invigorate your circulatory system, and are helpful in cases of muscular strains, colds, and infections.
➤ A gush for the arms
Direct the stream of water to the outside of your right arm, starting at the back of your hand and going up to your shoulder; then direct the water to the inside of your arm, from the shoulder down to your palm. Do the same with your left arm.
➤ A gush for the legs
Direct the stream of water to your right leg, starting at the front of your right foot and proceeding to the knee, then going downward along the back of your leg to the sole of your foot. Follow the same procedure with your left leg.

Pastor Kneipp rediscovered water treatment. He first tried the various procedures out on himself, with success.

Water treatments as well as plenty of sunshine and fresh air are important for keeping your body healthy.

➤ A gush for the face
Circle the stream of water over your face.

Treading Water

➤ Fill the bathtub with cold water, so that the water will reach just up to your fibula.
➤ Tread in the water in place.
➤ Alternating, lift one leg and then the other out of the water.

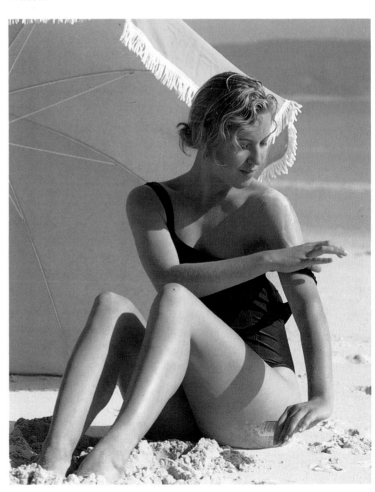

Too much sun is unhealthy, so avoid "baking" in the sun for too long. And always, even when you are in the shade, use a sun-block lotion with a high protection factor.

➤ If you are becoming too cold, get out of the bathtub and run around a bit.
➤ If you go to sleep right after treading water, you will have a restful sleep.

Air and Sun

Exposing your entire body to the air and sunbathing will toughen your body gently. Light and warmth furthermore will support the formation of vitamin D in your body.

Get used to walking around naked for at least 5 minutes a day in a well-ventilated room (or outside). When taking a sunbath, you should protect your head from direct sunlight and you must not stay in the sun so long that ultraviolet rays can harm your skin. Start by taking a sunbath for 5 minutes, and gradually increase the time to 30 minutes. Afterward, a cold shower is recommended.

Plants for Purifying the Skin

➤ Wild pansies
Tea from wild pansies (*Viola tricolor*) has a diaphoretic effect, cleans the blood, and is helpful in treating acne. (See sidebar.)
➤ Elderberry blossoms
Tea from elderberry (*Sambucus nigra*) blossoms has a reputation for inducing perspiration. It is helpful for treating colds accompanied by fever and for treating rheumatism. It also is used as a preventive measure to strengthen resistance. This tea is a diaphoretic, cleans the blood, and is helpful in treating impurities of the skin and bad body odor. (See sidebar.)
➤ Burdock root
Tea from burdock (*Articum lappa*) root is a diaphoretic and helps eliminate water from tissue. It also is used for rheumatism and gout, as well as for afflictions of the liver and gallbladder. (See sidebar.)

Tea from Wild Pansies
Gather the blooming plant and dry it. Pour ¼ liter (or quart) of hot water over 2 teaspoons of the plant, and let steep for 10 minutes. Drink 1 cup three times a day for several weeks.

Tea from Elderberry Blossoms
Pour ¼ liter (or quart) of boiling water over 3 teaspoons of elderberry blossoms, steep for 10 minutes, and strain. Drink 1 very hot cup of the tea three times a day.

Tea from Burdock Root
Pour ¼ liter (or quart) of cold water over 3 teaspoons of the cut-up root. Steep for 5 hours. Then bring to a boil, cook for 1 minute, and strain. Drink 1 cup three times a day. Also, dab the tea on the afflicted area of the skin.

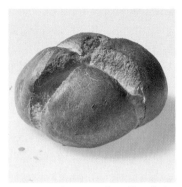

A cure with milk rolls by F. X. Mayr is one of the most effective fasts you can do.

Methods of Fasting and Partial Fasting

"The best of all medicines are fasting and diets. You just have to apply them correctly."—Dr. F. X. Mayr, Styrian physician and inventor of the milk roll cure, 1875–1965

Complete fasting, which means not eating any solid food, is one of the most effective methods of detoxification. But you don't necessarily have to avoid food completely in order to help your body to detoxify. A positive cleansing effect also will be achieved if days of total fasting are alternated with days when you are only fasting part of the day. Two or three total-fasting days, when you will be taking in only fluids (drinking days), are followed by two or three days of partial fasting (eating days), when vegetarian food (fruit, potatoes, rice, and so forth) is allowed. Toward the end of the cure, food intake gradually is increased.

When you fast, your body switches to "inner food intake," which means that reserves are used. Many impurities and toxins are thereby eliminated.

Deep Cleansing—Fasting Cures

Nourishment from the Inside

Normally, the organism receives its energy from nutrients taken in from the outside. However, when fasting, a shift to the inner nutrients takes place. The body uses its inner reserves. In this process, no muscles, nerves, or vital organs are used at first, although impurities and toxins are flushed out.

Fasting Cures Are Drinking Cures

While fasting, the body's supply of animal and vegetable protein, fat, and carbohydrates is largely stopped. The body, nevertheless, needs vital foods, vitamins, minerals, and trace elements. These are taken in liquid form with diluted fruit juices, vegetable broths, teas, or whey products.

During a fast, drinking must not be stopped. In fact, fasting cures are always drinking cures. The liquids will transport loosened toxins and waste products from the body by means of the intestines, the skin, and the kidneys.

Unburdening and Cleansing the Intestines

The intestines, especially, which are always in use, will be unburdened over the duration of a fast. For a while, the intestines will not have to take in food and can tend to their second task, which is the elimination of by-products from the metabolism.

Because the intestines do not empty out on their own, when fasting we have to assist them by using Epsom salt (magnesium sulfate), Glauber salt (sodium sulfate), or enemas. Otherwise, the danger exists that a renewed toxicity will be spread from the intestines.

During detoxification, it's advisable to drink every two days a glass of a Glauber- or Epsom-salt solution, or take an enema every second day. The salt solutions have the advantage of flushing the intestines completely from top to bottom. Thereby, incrustations of food still contained in the intestines will be dissolved and washed out. An enema, on the other hand, will cleanse mainly the lower part of the intestines.

While you fast, it is important to drink a lot of liquid to eliminate toxins. Otherwise, a fasting crisis, due to a renewed poisoning, could occur.

Soup for Fasting
(for 4 Portions)
Ingredients
100 g (3½ oz.) celery root,
100 g parsley root, 100 g
fennel root, 50 g (1¾ oz.)
potatoes, 30 g (1 oz.) leaks,
1 small carrot, some grains
of sea salt, yeast flakes, 2
bay leaves, 4 juniper berries,
4 peppercorns, and 1 liter
(or qt.) water.

Preparation
Peel and cut vegetables, and
place in cold water. Add the
spices, and bring to a boil;
allow to simmer over low
heat for 20 to 30 minutes.
Strain, and add salt and
¼ teaspoon of yeast flakes to
season.

If you don't have much time,
you can cook this soup by
using vegetable powder or
cubes. Because of their high
salt content, dilute more
strongly than indicated.

A Day of Fasting, Devised by Dr. Otto Buchinger

➤ *Morning:* Cleanse your intestines by using Epsom or Glauber salts or an enema; afterward, have a cup of unsweetened peppermint tea.

➤ *Breakfast:* Have 2 cups of herbal tea (rosemary, peppermint, mallow, ginseng) or diluted black tea—add a teaspoon of honey, if desired.

➤ *Mid-morning:* Drink 2 glasses of mineral water or 2 cups of fruit or herbal tea.

➤ *Lunch:* Have ¼ liter (or quart) of vegetable broth (soup for fasting—see sidebar) or ⅛ liter (or quart) of fresh vegetable juice mixed with the same amount of mineral water (either hot or cold).

➤ *Afternoon:* Have 2 cups of herbal or fruit tea with lemon and/or half a teaspoon of honey.

➤ *Dinner:* Drink ⅛ liter (or quart) of fruit or vegetable juice diluted with the same amount of mineral water or vegetable broth.

How to Cleanse Your Intestines

➤ Stir a teaspoon of Epsom or Glauber salts into ¼ liter (or quart) of lukewarm water.

➤ To improve the taste, add a few drops of lemon.

➤ Drink the solution in small gulps in the morning on an empty stomach.

➤ Afterward, drink unsweetened peppermint tea or some juice.

➤ Because you will soon need to empty your bowels, stay near a bathroom.

➤ As an alternative, it might be sufficient to simply drink a glass of buttermilk, whey, or sauerkraut juice in the morning on an empty stomach.

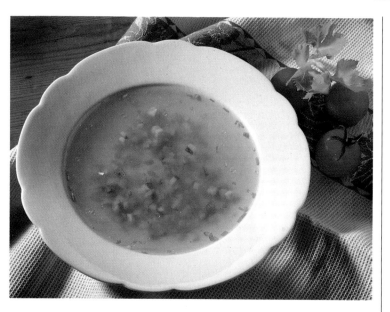

The soup for fasting is a hearty, well-seasoned vegetable soup—a delicious enrichment on a day of fasting.

➤ *Before bedtime:* To relax, have a cup of herbal tea (valerian or chamomile).
➤ *In-between times:* Drink as much mineral water as you like, at least 2 liters (or quarts).

Schedule for a Juice Day

➤ *Morning:* To cleanse your intestines, Epsom or Glauber salts in lukewarm water, or an enema with 2 cups of rosemary tea for stimulation.
➤ *Breakfast:* Drink 60 grams (or about 2 ounces) of both fruit juice and vegetable juice, and 30 grams (about 1 ounce) of herbal juice (freshly squeezed or bought at a health food store), diluted with the same amount of mineral water.
➤ *Mid-morning:* The same as for Breakfast.
➤ *Lunch:* The same as for Breakfast.
➤ *Afternoon:* The same as for Breakfast.
➤ *Dinner:* The same as for Breakfast.
➤ *Before bedtime:* A cup of valerian tea for relaxation.

TIP
Avoid leeks, onions, and kale, as they cause flatulence.

➤ *In-between times:* As much mineral water as desired, at least 2 liters (or quarts).

A Fasting Cure with Whey

This fasting cure is a drinking cure with whey (diet whey), herbal juices, and herbal teas. It is especially well suited for:

➤ Constipation
➤ Food poisoning
➤ Skin problems
➤ Chronic liver diseases
➤ Preventive detoxification and purification

Its effect is based on a thorough cleansing of the intestines and an unburdening of the liver and gallbladder.

Dextrorotatory Lactic Acid

The advantage of a cure with diet whey has to do with whey containing dextrorotatory lactic acid, which will be used immediately during metabolism and thus no detrimental overacidification will occur. This protective type of fasting can be done easily while working.

What You Should Drink

For this cure, take 1 to 1½ liters (or quarts) of whey low in protein (available at the health food store) in five to seven portions, and 5 tablespoons of juices made from fresh plants (especially artichokes, nettles, and dandelion) 1 tablespoon at a time throughout the day.

Start your day with a Glauber- or Epsom-salt solution (or an enema). For breakfast, drink herbal tea or diluted black tea with a teaspoon of honey. In the evening, drink 2 cups of green oats tea (from the health food store), which will work as an additional diuretic, as well as stimulate digestion and the production of uric acid and other products of metabolism.

You can make whey from whey curds and then mix it with fruit juice. Whey curds can be bought at health food stores.

A Whey Drink
Mix whey curds with freshly pressed juice from oranges, grapefruit, lemon, or buckthorn.

Various Partial-Fasting Programs

Partial-fasting programs are based mainly on mono-diets, whereby intake of food is restricted to the consumption of a few foods—for the most part, vegetarian food and milk products.

Such mono-diets are well suited for healthy people as preventive purification and detoxification measures, but they also are recommended for individuals suffering from obesity, digestive and skin problems, or unfavorable blood counts. However, if mono-diets are extended for more than three to four weeks, deficiencies can occur.

The Milk Roll Cure, Devised by F. X. Mayr

Definition: A soothing diet based on whole milk and aged wheat rolls (cure rolls) in conjunction with special training for chewing.

Especially useful for: People suffering from chronic digestive complaints, obesity, problems of toxicity, or gastritis.

Effects: Unburdening the digestive tract, special training for the saliva glands, detoxifying the body, and normalizing uric-acid and blood counts.

What you may eat daily: As many aged rolls until you are satiated and up to half a liter (or quart) of milk. At noon, some vegetable broth; in the evening, 1 to 2 cups of herbal tea with a teaspoon of honey swallowed in small amounts from a teaspoon. The rolls are dried in the open for two to four days before consumption.

Liquids: Mineral water and diluted herbal teas, at least 2 liters (or quarts) daily.

This is how you eat (training for correct chewing):
➤ Cut the dried roll into of finger-width slices.
➤ Bite off a small piece, and chew consciously and without haste until the bite becomes almost liquefied.

Wheat rolls and milk: these are the mainstay of the soothing diet developed by F. X. Mayr.

➤ Then sip a teaspoon of milk from the spoon, continue chewing, and finally swallow the bite.

➤ Take the next bite. To eat a single roll should take you nearly half an hour.

➤ Stop eating as soon as you feel slightly full (don't eat the rest of the rolls and the milk).

Advantages: The training for chewing invigorates atrophied saliva glands and teaches us to eat correctly again—that is, slowly and not too much. Furthermore, the Mayr cure is an extremely soothing cure for the stomach and intestines.

The Potato Diet

Definition: A mono-diet that drains excessive water from the body, mainly consisting of potatoes, without salt.

Especially useful for: People who suffer from elevated uric-acid counts, obesity, gout, or rheumatism.

Effects: Diuretic, lowers blood cholesterol, unburdens the metabolism, digestion, and blood circulation, counteracts hyperacidity of the body, and removes accumulated water from connective tissue.

What you may eat daily: Two pounds of potatoes (in their skin), in five to seven portions, other vegetables, and ¼ liter (or quart) of vegetable broth.

Preparation: Cook potatoes in their skin to conserve their mineral content, and eat potatoes with their skin with a bit of butter, some yeast flakes, and shredded raw vegetables or cooked vegetables (tomatoes, carrots, black radishes, parsley root, chicory) or low-fat quark with herbs. (Quark is a kind of cheese product similar to a cross between yogurt and small-curd cottage cheese.)

Liquids: At least 2 liters (or quarts) of mineral water, diluted fruit and vegetable juices, and vegetable broth (see sidebar on page 89 for recipe).

Tip: How about trying a potato facial mask? Mash

In cases of rheumatism, gout, and obesity, a potato diet often is a miracle cure. If you like potatoes, why don't you try it?

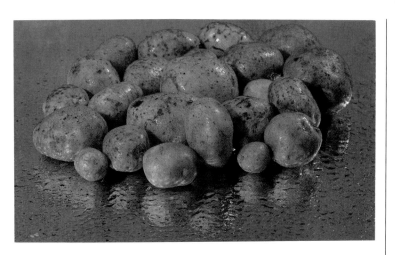

Potatoes are a good choice for a mono-diet, and a face mask made from potatoes gives you health and beauty at the same time.

half a boiled peeled potato, mix in the yolk of an egg, and add a few drops of cream. Cover your face with the mask for 20 minutes. Wash it off with lukewarm water. Your skin will be so smooth that you won't need to apply any moisturizing cream afterward.

The Carrot Diet

Definition: A mono-diet that is rich in minerals and fiber.

Especially useful for: People with frequent inflammation of the mucous membrane of the stomach and the intestines.

Effects: Removes accumulated water, soothes the intestines.

What you may eat daily: Carrots—2 to 3 pounds in five to seven portions.

Preparation: Eat the carrots raw, shredded, or cooked briefly. Always add a little bit of oil, because carrots contain a precursor of vitamin A that is soluble in fat. Season with fresh herbs and spices, but avoid salt. Eat a portion of potatoes in their skins at noon or in the evening to accompany the carrot diet.

The Rice Diet

Definition: A mono-diet consisting mostly of unprocessed rice.

Especially useful for: People with circulatory problems, high blood pressure, and water retention in their connective tissue.

Effects: Unburdening the circulatory system, lowering blood pressure, flushing out excess water, and cleansing the connective tissue.

What you may eat daily: About 200 to 300 grams (7 to 10½ ounces) of unprocessed rice, prepared without salt, in five to seven portions, half a liter (or quart) of vegetable broth (see sidebar on page 89), apples, and vegetables.

Preparation: In the morning, prepare the rice as milk rice with a bit of cinnamon, and eat it with some baked apples or applesauce. At noon, boil the rice in water or broth, and eat it with some steamed tomatoes, chicory, or other vegetables, seasoned with yeast flakes, a little butter, and fresh herbs.

The Fruit Diet

Definition: A fat- and protein-free mono-diet consisting mainly of fresh fruit.

Especially well suited for: Obesity, overconsumption of meat, a lack of vitamins, a poor blood count, circulatory problems, and edema.

Effects: Unburdening the metabolism, lowering uric-acid count and cholesterol, decreasing excess protein, and getting rid of water in the body.

What you may eat daily: Fruit—2 to 3 pounds, in five to seven portions.

➤ Try the combination recommended by Professor Heupke: About 400 grams (14 ounces) of apples, 700

Whether a carrot or rice diet or a fruit day, these partial-fasting programs help you to purify your system. But you should not stay on these programs for too long.

The Healing Properties of Various Fruit

Apples	Shredded: for diarrhea or constipation; eaten whole: for light headaches, hangover, lowering of cholesterol, prevention of hardening of the arteries
Blueberries	Accelerate healing of wounds, lowering of uric-acid count
Sour cherries	Antirheumatic, diuretic, blood cleansing
Black currants	Antirheumatic, and for high blood pressure and lowering of cholesterol
Red currants	For constipation, soothing of pain
Elderberries	For prevention of infectious diseases, lowering of uric-acid count, bronchitis
Gooseberries	For constipation and exhaustion
Grapes	Strengthening of the heart, stimulation of the circulatory system, blood cleansing
Peaches	For clear skin
Pears	For diarrhea, increase in brain capacity
Plums	For nervousness and sleep disorders
Strawberries	Cleansing of the skin and the blood, and for a slight headache

"Your food shall be your medicine, your medicine shall be your food." (Hippocrates, 4th century B.C.)

grams (24½ ounces) of pears, and 400 grams of bananas.
➤ Especially important fruit for metabolism and digestion are pineapple, papayas, and bananas.
➤ If you want to eat something warm at noon or at night, you can eat potatoes in their skin along with the fruit.
➤ Six walnuts a day provide important B vitamins, polyene acid, and vitamin E.

The Wheat Diet

Definition: Mono-diet consisting mainly of whole-wheat bran enriched with fiber, protein, fatty acids, vitamins, and minerals (preparation available at health food stores).

Especially useful for: People who want to detoxify, or to reduce their weight or maintain it.

Effects: Cleansing of the gastrointestinal tract, elimination of water, and unburdening of the heart and circulatory system.

What you may eat daily: About 200 grams (7 ounces) of whole-wheat diet preparation in five to seven portions, fresh fruit, cooked vegetables, yogurt.

Preparation: Per portion, stir 5 tablespoons of wheat diet preparation into about 12 tablespoons of cold or hot water, and season with yogurt, fresh fruit, or cooked vegetables (for more recipes, consult the back of the package).

➤ Piquant wheat diet: Cook 100 grams (3½ ounces) of champignons (an edible fungus) in a bit of water, and about 12 tablespoons of instant vegetable broth. Add 5 tablespoons of wheat diet, and season with half a teaspoon of yeast flakes and some cooking herbs.

➤ Wheat diet breakfast: Stir ⅛ liter (or quart) of water into a container of low-fat yogurt, stir in 5 tablespoons of whole-wheat diet, and serve on a plate with a quarter of a shredded apple, shredded lemon peel (organic), 100 grams (about 3½ ounces) of sliced banana, and six grapes.

A Day of Uncooked Food, Devised by Dr. Bircher-Brenner

Definition: A diet based on fresh vegetarian food ("refreshing food for life"—Dr. Bircher-Brenner), consisting of raw fruits and vegetables and muesli.

How about a wheat muesli with yogurt and fresh fruit for breakfast? With such a breakfast, you will feel fit and vigorous throughout the day.

Especially useful for: Obesity, all digestive problems like constipation, intestinal infections, and so forth.

Effects: Because of the high content of fiber and pectin in whole wheat, vegetables, and fruit, these foods are better for digestion than other foods. What's more, you are chewing for a longer time and using more saliva, and thus you are satiated sooner and eat less.

This is what you may eat daily: In the morning, a Bircher muesli (see sidebar); at noon, a plate with raw vegetables and fruit with a light dressing; in the evening, the same as at noon.

Preparation: The vegetables usually are eaten raw or only cooked slightly. Raw plants contain natural antibiotics, vital mineral salts, vitamins, and enzymes.

Liquids: Tea, especially rose hip tea, and mineral water.

The Milk and Vegetable Diet

Definition: A diet consisting of plants and milk products that is low in protein and fat (which means low in calories).

Especially useful for: Older individuals, for an extended period of time (not a mono-diet).

Effect: Rejuvenating the cell potential.

What you may eat daily: About 30 grams (2 tablespoons) of various high-quality cold-pressed oils like germ, kernel, or seed oil (linseed, thistle, sunflower, or corn oil), 10 grams (less than ½ ounce) of butter, 200 grams (7 ounces) of grains, 300 grams (10½ ounces) of whole-wheat bread, 600 grams (21 ounces) of various vegetables and fruit (raw or cooked), legumes only once in a while (for example, peas, beans, and lentils), and 300 to 400 grams (10½ to 14 ounces) of milk, yogurt, kefir, or whey or 30 grams (2 tablespoons) of Harz or Mainz cheese, 50 grams (1¾ ounces) of low-

Bircher muesli, the original muesli by Bircher-Brenner, is the classic among the muesli varieties. It has a high-fiber content, so it is especially good for the intestines.

An advantage of the diet based on milk products and vegetables is that hyperacidity of tissues, a common side effect of many diets and fasting cures, will rarely occur.

Regardless of whether you are on a partial-fasting program or doing a complete fast, it is important to drink large quantities of liquids. Blossom and herbal teas are especially well suited.

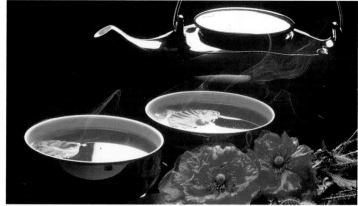

fat quark, or 70 grams (2½ ounces) of baker's cheese (Hüttenkäse). How you would like to combine these foods and eat them during the day is up to you.

What you should avoid: All products directly derived from animals, like meat, fish, and eggs.

Tips for Total and Partial Fasting

These are some supplementary measures you can take on a complete or a partial fast:

➤ Every second day, cleanse your intestines with Epsom salt or an enema.

➤ Drink at least 2 to 3 liters (or quarts) a day (include the liquid meals): noncarbonated mineral water; diluted tea from blossoms, roots, fruit, and herbs; diluted fruit and vegetable juices.

➤ Move around a lot. The minimum is one fast-paced walk a day.

➤ Take especially good care of your body. You might want to take a bath with increasing temperatures, give yourself a dry-brush massage, or visit the sauna or the steam bath. They will all support detoxification.

➤ Refrain as much as possible from alcohol and nicotine.

➤ Regard every meal (even though it might consist only

If you don't have time or you have no desire to undergo a complete fasting cure, why not start with a partial fast for one day?

of liquids) as a true meal, and sit down at a nicely set table. Sip your fasting drink with a spoon, or drink it slowly in small gulps.

➤ After lunch, lie down with a hot-water bottle on your stomach. This will make detoxification easier for your liver.

A Regular Day of Fasting

If you undertake a day of partial or complete fasting once a week or every two weeks, in the long run you will achieve very good purifying results and prevent obesity and all its dangerous ramifications. It is important that you fast *regularly*, however. It is better, for example, to fast once a month on a certain day than to fast more frequently but irregularly.

Try Fridays

As a day of purification, Fridays seem ideal for many people. Eating little and consciously on Friday will make it unlikely that you will overeat on the weekend, which otherwise could be the case. In other respects too, you will be able to harness more restraint, and you will become more aware of your body and experience nature more intensely.

From a Day of Fasting to a Short Cure

It will have positive effects if you extend your regular day of purification to a short cure once in a while. This way, you just have to lengthen the fast by a few days.

On such a short cure, you should cleanse your intestines every second day. If you undertake only a single day of purification, it is not imperative to cleanse your intestines, although the procedure is always beneficial. Cleaning out your intestines also alleviates the feeling of being hungry.

Try out different one-day fasts. Soon you will find the one that works best for you.

Friday is the optimal day for fasting. The monks back in the Middle Ages knew this.

TIP
A single day of purification after a holiday filled with rich meals is a respite for your body and soul.

75

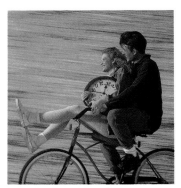

It is important to plan your week of fasting according to an exact time schedule.

Within a single week, you will have purified your body and made it healthy again. The program presented here is your personal adviser for a week of fasting.

Program for a Week of Purification

Exactly What Is Involved?

During a week of purification, all five organs of elimination (including the liver and gallbladder) need to be stimulated at the same time. This is accomplished by fasting or partial fasting, whereby certain foods and/or beverages are consumed that have tissue-cleansing, diuretic, and purifying properties. In addition, further measures of purification are used.

Your Personal Adviser for a Week of Purification

Everything you will need to know for all seven days of a week of fasting is covered here. All important questions are discussed, such as:

➤ What is the structure of the week of purification?
➤ Who should undertake a week of purification?
➤ When is the best time for it?
➤ How frequently can it be repeated?

In detailed plans for every day, you will find menus, tables of nutrition, and practical tips. And you will get the original recipe for the muesli developed by Dr. Max Bircher-Brenner.

The Organs of Elimination at a Glance

ORGAN FOR DETOXIFICATION	ELIMINATION VIA	MEASURES OF DETOXIFICATION
Intestines	Stool	Fasting or partial fasting, saline solutions (or enemas), extensive chewing of food
Kidneys	Urine	Drinking a lot of fluids, fasting, foods that cleanse tissue during partial fasting (for example, potatoes and rice), diuretic teas
Liver	Stool, urine, sweat	Fasting or partial fasting, rest, warmth
Lungs	Exhaling nasal and bronchial secretions	Physical activity, exhaling forcefully, singing
Skin	Sweat	Treatments with hot and cold water, diaphoretic measures, massage

This chart gives you an overview of the purification capabilities of the five organs of elimination.

Plan for a Week of Purification

➤ You will start with two days of a liquid fast.
➤ Three days of a partial fast will follow (eating days).
➤ At the end, there will be two days of buildup.

Before starting, some questions regarding your suitability for fasting should be answered.

Important Questions Before You Begin

Who May Undertake a Week of Purification?

Who may do a week of purification? When should you do it and how often? Here, you will find comprehensive information.

This program is appropriate for all people who are healthy and would like to undertake some preventive measures for the upkeep of their health, as well as to generally purify and regenerate their body. But a week of purification also has proven to be very effective in treating a number of ailments, such as skin problems, muscle tension, depression, digestive problems (acid indigestion, constipation), obesity, and high uric-acid or cholesterol counts. However, anyone who is seriously ill and under the care of a physician, takes medications regularly, or has any kind of misgivings should consult a physician beforehand.

When Is the Best Time to Do It?

Start the cure when it is convenient for you. For people who are employed, it is best to start the cure on a Saturday. This way, the two days of liquid fasting, which do require an adjustment by your body, will be on the weekend.

You don't have to stick to the schedule religiously. If you take well to the two days of liquid fasting, you may add another day. However, it is important that on the two days of buildup, you gradually and carefully increase your food intake. You don't want to go from a partial fast to eating pork roast with dumplings immediately.

How Frequently Can This Cure Be Repeated?

It is useful to repeat a week of purification several times a year. It would make sense, for example, to do it at the beginning of each season, especially at the beginning of spring. This is the time of year when your metabolism is adjusting to warmer days, and toxins and fat deposits acquired during the winter should be eliminated.

Schedule and Guidelines for All Seven Days

➤ On the first morning of the week of purification, drink water with Epsom or Glauber salt (or have an enema). On the third, fifth, and sixth mornings, it's advised to cleanse your intestines with one of these methods again. However, if you have too frequent bowel movements or even diarrhea, then restrict your cleansing measures.

➤ The more effectively the individual organs for detoxification are included in the treatment plan, the better the results of the purification will be.

➤ For every day of the week, plan a detoxification measure via the skin—for example, a sauna or steam bath, Kneipp's gushes, or a bath with increasing temperatures.

➤ Every morning, do a dry-brush massage and expose yourself to fresh air.

➤ For every day, plan outdoor exercises for the elimination of gaseous toxins by means of the lungs, such as swimming, bicycling, or playing tennis. Overdress to induce perspiration, and wear clothing made from natural fiber. Don't forget to wash off the perspiration afterward with warm water. If you take a walk, walk briskly, which will induce deeper breathing and lead to an increase of oxygen in the tissue. If you feel weak on liquid-fast days, then reduce your exercises, but don't eliminate all physical activity.

➤ If possible, rest for an hour after the noon meal; this also will stimulate the liver. Place a hot-water bottle

The results of a week of purification depend a great deal on correct planning. Try to include all organs for toxic elimination.

against your stomach. When lying down, the blood supply in the liver increases by 40 percent.

➤ Don't drink any alcohol during these seven days. Limit your use of tobacco. If you can't or don't want to do without coffee, you may drink a cup in the morning, but without milk or sugar.

➤ During the entire fast, make sure you drink a lot of liquid.

Fasting days, days of eating, days of buildup—here, you can find everything you will need to know for a week of purification.

First and Second Days—the Days of Fasting

➤ Buchinger, juice, or whey fast. Decide which one you want to use. (Refer to the previous chapter for the specifics of each fast.)

➤ Fasting days are days for drinking. You may drink more than the amounts indicated for the fast. Drinking is also helpful if you are feeling hungry.

➤ If you find yourself experiencing circulatory problems, brew yourself a cup of black tea and add half a teaspoon of honey. However, don't drink this too late at night, or you might not be able to sleep. A glass of buttermilk is helpful for alleviating dizziness and weakness.

Third to Fifth Day—the Days of Eating

➤ Choose one of the partial fasts (described in the previous chapter) and stay with the particular diet for three days.

➤ Every day, drink a cup of tea made from birch leaves, nettle, or juniper berries to cleanse the blood and eliminate water from the tissues.

Sixth and Seventh Days—the Days of Buildup

The days of buildup are used to get your body acquainted with normal food once more. The intestines, in par-

Buildup Day During a Week of Purification

General Guidelines

➤ Continue to eat little as before. As soon as you feel slightly satiated, stop eating.

➤ Eat slowly and chew thoroughly. This way, you will feel satiated sooner. Drink a lot of liquid (herbal teas and mineral water).

What You May Eat on Days of Buildup

➤ Bread and rolls, as well as linseed and soaked prunes or figs for stimulation of digestion

➤ Cooked vegetables or vegetable soup

➤ Raw food in easy-to-digest salads and vegetables dishes

➤ Buttermilk, yogurt, curdled milk, low-fat milk, or low-fat quark, some butter, perhaps a soft-boiled egg, some lean ham or turkey breast

What You Should Still Avoid

➤ Legumes (peas, beans, lentils) and all varieties of cooked cabbage

➤ Fatty foods, including everything that is fried and breaded

➤ Meat, sausages, organ meats, and dishes containing gravy

➤ Sweets, including, ice-cream and chocolate

➤ Stimulants, like coffee and alcohol

What you may eat during the days of buildup, as well as what you should avoid, can be found in the chart above.

ticular, must gradually get accustomed to having more food come in from the outside.

Be careful not to overburden the intestines now, because cramps, stomach trouble, or malaise could be the outcome. Furthermore, your hard-won results of purification could quickly disappear.

However, if you are in tune with your body, you won't be craving heavy meals after five days of reduced-food intake.

TIP
On the sixth day, before breakfast, you may want to have an enema to clean out your intestines.

Meal Plan for the Sixth Day

Breakfast: A slice of whole-wheat bread or two slices of crisp bread with some butter, an apple, and 2 cups of herbal or black tea.

Lunch: Thick potato-vegetable soup (for recipe, see page 31), a small container of yogurt with a teaspoon of buckthorn juice, and herbal tea.

Dinner: Two slices of crisp bread with a little butter, some quark with herbs, a glass of buttermilk with a teaspoon of linseed oil, and herbal tea.

Meal Plan for the Seventh Day

Breakfast: Bircher muesli (see receipt below) and 2 cups of herbal tea.

Lunch: A plate of raw, easy-to-digest salads and vegetables, along with potatoes in their skin or potatoes with cumin, some lean ham or turkey breast, and herbal tea. (For tips on preparing raw food, see opposite page.)

Dinner: Two slices of whole-wheat bread or rolls with a little bit of butter and some quark or baker's cheese, or quark with fresh herbs, or a soft-boiled egg or a small container of yogurt with a teaspoon of linseed, and herbal tea.

This is the original Bircher muesli recipe.

Recipe for the Original Bircher Muesli

Mix a container of low-fat yogurt (or a cup of milk) with 2 to 3 tablespoons of oats, a small shredded apple, a teaspoon of chopped nuts, a teaspoon of honey (or soaked raisins), and fresh lemon juice. You can choose the nuts and the fruit you want, and you could replace the oats with other flakes, wheat germ, or freshly ground grains (soaked overnight).

More Tips for the Seventh Day—Preparation of Raw Food, According to Dr. Bircher-Brenner

For a plate of raw food, all ingredients need to be washed well, so that they can be taken up by the intestines under optimal conditions. You should cut the food as follows.

➤ Grate: Red beets, black radish, celery root, carrots, kohlrabi, daikon, parsley root
➤ Cut into thin slices (shred): All varieties of cabbage and kale (white cabbage, red cabbage, Chinese cabbage, kohlrabi, etc.), fennel, cucumber, celery, endive, spinach, radish (or leave whole), zucchini
➤ Cut into somewhat larger slices: Peppers, endive, chicory
➤ Slice: Tomatoes
➤ Do not cut: Boston lettuce, cress

During a single meal, it's best not to eat more than three kinds of vegetables. Season your raw food with a dressing made from high-grade kernel, germ, or seed oil, or use yogurt, lemon, fresh herbs (chives, parsley, basil, dill), a bit of onion, raw garlic, yeast flakes, and spices (no salt).

Unsaturated Fatty Acids Are Good for You

The unsaturated fatty acids in vegetable oils can prevent hardening of the arteries and invigorate circulation.

On the other hand, saturated fatty acids—for example, in meat, sausage, and eggs—are the main reason for an elevated cholesterol count, and consequently the cause of vascular constriction. Avoid foods high in cholesterol.

Depending on the kind of vegetable, grating, shredding, or slicing is recommended.

Light Yogurt Dressing for Raw Vegetables
Mix 3 tablespoons of yogurt, 1 teaspoon of lemon juice, and 1 to 2 teaspoons of fresh diced herbs.

Oil Dressing for Raw Vegetables
Mix 3 tablespoons of high-grade oil, 1 teaspoon of lemon juice, and 1 to 2 teaspoons of finely cut herbs.

You will find tips for selecting vegetables on this list. If you follow the guidelines for buying, storing, and preparing food, you will do your body a lot of good.

Be Alert When Going Shopping

When buying and preparing food, you should be aware of the following:

➤ Select ripe fruit and vegetables, if possible, organically grown. Eat about 300 grams (10½ ounces) of fruit and vegetables a day. If you eat a great deal of raw food at night though, you will run the risk of too many toxins of fermentation forming in your intestines.

➤ Buy mostly locally grown fruit in season. However, for enrichment, imported fruit are of some value. Fresh papayas and pineapple contain proteolytic enzymes, which are helpful for the digestion of meat. Bananas have a positive effect on the large intestines. Kiwis contain a large amount of vitamin C.

➤ Avoid fruit grown in hothouses.

➤ It's best not to store fruit and vegetables for more than 48 hours.

➤ Wash fruit and vegetables thoroughly, but only for a short time.

➤ Because many vital substances are stored in the skin, washing is often preferable to peeling.

➤ Cut up fruit and vegetables only a short time before using them. As soon as the surface of shredded or cut fruit and vegetables comes into contact with warmth and oxygen, important vital substances are lost.

➤ Cook vegetables for as short a time as possible. Thus, nutrients and taste are preserved.

➤ Fresh herbs contain many vitamins and minerals. They are a superior seasoning, because they enhance the taste of food. You will also need less salt.

➤ People who use herbs instead of salt for seasoning protect themselves from high blood pressure.

➤ Instead of regular table salt, use sea salt, because, besides natrium chloride, it also contains numerous important minerals.

➤ Add a bit of fresh garlic to your raw-vegetable dressing. It fights infections, stimulates gastric fluids, and can dissolve urinary crystals. Furthermore, since antiquity, garlic has been known for its rejuvenating properties, and it will prevent hardening of the arteries.

➤ Make it a rule to consume half of your food raw—for example, fruit, grain, vegetables, nuts, herbs, and whole milk.

Fresh garden herbs not only taste good, but they also are good for you. Take advantage of the natural healing properties from your garden.

Fresh Garden Herbs and Their Effects

Chervil	For flatulence, stimulating, rich in iron
Chives	Stimulates appetite
Dill	Helps digestion, prevents bloating
Lemongrass	Stimulates digestion, diaphoretic, soothes cramps
Marjoram	Soothes cramps, is calming on the stomach
Mint	Stimulant, rich in iron
Parsley	Stimulating, invigorating
Pimpernel	Stimulates appetite and digestion
Rosemary	Strengthens the stomach
Sage	Stimulates digestion, for flatulence
Tarragon	Stimulates appetite, helpful for stomach complaints and rheumatism

TIP
Coriander, anise, and fennel are effective herbs for flatulence.

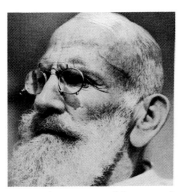

The inventor of the original Bircher muesli, Dr. Bircher-Brenner is also known for his views on nutrition and lifestyle.

Dr. Bircher-Brenner's detoxification cure is useful for all kinds of complaints that result from eating too much food and unhealthy food.

Dr. Bircher-Brenner's Seven-Day Detoxification Cure

"Every bit of unnecessary food weakens you. It does not make you stronger, as is often assumed. It is not an asset to your health, but impairs it."—Dr. Max Bircher-Brunner, Swiss physician and specialist in nutrition 1867–1939

Benefits of Fruit, Vegetables, and Grain

The detoxification cure developed by Dr. Bircher-Brunner has proven to be helpful for all symptoms produced from eating too much food and food of low quality. Such symptoms include irritability, exhaustion, and stomach problems. You can conduct this detoxification cure several times a year.

On this diet, it is preferable to eat fruit and vegetables in season. Many properties contained in vegetables and fruit strengthen the immune system, fight viruses, and protect us from the dangers of free radicals. Aggressive oxygen molecules, free radicals harm the body's cells and weaken the immune system. The high-fiber content in fruit, vegetables, and whole-kernel grains bind the cholesterol in the intestines so that it can't get into the bloodstream.

During this seven-day cure, practically no salt should be used; furthermore, strong seasonings and sweets should be avoided, as should alcohol and tobacco.

Meal Plan for the Week

The Course of the Cure

The week of the cure starts with three days of raw food, followed by two days of a mixed diet and finally two days of buildup.

Meals Plan for First Three Days of Raw Food

Breakfast: Bircher muesli (see page 82 for original recipe) with wheat germ and fresh fruit in season, 2 cups of rose hip tea.

   Lunch: A plate with raw vegetables and salads (for example, celery root, tomatoes, cucumber, lettuces, cress, parsley root, and red turnips—but, if possible, no more than three varieties of vegetables per serving), herbal tea.

   Dinner: Bircher muesli (see Breakfast).

   Rose hips have a slightly diuretic and purgative effect, because they contain numerous fruit acids and pectins. This is why they are recommended as a tea. (To prepare the tea, see the sidebar.)

Meal Plan for Next Two Days of a Mixed Diet

Breakfast: Bircher muesli with wheat germ, two slices of whole-kernel bread with a bit of butter or plant-based margarine, rose hip tea.

   Lunch: Vegetable broth (see recipe in sidebar on page 89), a plate of fresh fruit and raw vegetables (radish, green beans, lettuce), potatoes in their skin with a bit of butter, herbal tea.

   Dinner: See Breakfast.

Meal Plan for Final Two Days of Buildup

Breakfast: Bircher muesli, two slices of whole-kernel bread, yogurt with a teaspoon of buckthorn, rose hip tea.

   Lunch: Vegetable broth (see recipe in sidebar on page

Rose Hip Tea
Pour ¼ liter (or quart) of water over 3 teaspoons of dried rose hips, bring to a boil, let boil for 10 minutes, and strain.

There are three different meal plans for this cure.

Pear Honey
Ingredients
Five large pears, 250 g (8¾ oz.) of forest or blossom honey, 2 tablespoons of a seasoning mixture (which you can buy from the Jura Company in Konstanz, Germany). This mixture contains 28 g (almost 1 oz.) of ground fennel root or spignel root, 24 g (a little more than ¾ oz.) of ground licorice root, and 22 g (about ¾ oz.) of ground stonecrop.

Preparation
Wash and quarter the pears, and remove their core. Cook them in a little water until they are soft; then strain and puree. While the pears are cooking, heat the honey in a double boiler until it becomes liquid. Then add 2 tablespoons of the ground-herb mixture and the pear sauce. Fill into jars with screw-on lids, and store in the refrigerator.

89), fresh fruit and raw vegetables (cauliflower, spinach, lettuce), steamed tomatoes, unprocessed rice with a bit of butter, or potatoes stuffed with quark and herbs (see recipe below), herbal tea.

Dinner: The same as for breakfast, but with marmalade on bread and honey in tea.

Further Tips and Recipes

The Advantages of the Bircher Muesli

If you eat Bircher muesli for breakfast, then you will be doing something good for your body and your mood. Bircher muesli contains the following:
➤ A great deal of calcium (from the milk)
➤ Sufficient fiber for your intestines
➤ Sufficient vitamins because of the fruit
➤ Strong healing effects due to the various fruit (see table on page 71)
➤ Many nutrients and minerals for your enzyme metabolism

With this breakfast, you not only will keep your intestines working, but you also will be provided with proteolytic enzymes, the necessary coenzymes in vitamin form, and thus will help your body to detoxify. The good taste of this muesli is a pleasant bonus.

Potatoes Filled with Quark and Herbs

Ingredients: Three fairly large potatoes, 200 grams (7 ounces) of low-fat quark, several teaspoons of milk, finely cut chives, and marjoram

Preparation: Bake potatoes in the oven at 225°C (435°F) for about 30 minutes, take them out, partially scoop them out, and fill them with the quark mixture (stir the herbs and milk into the low-fat quark).

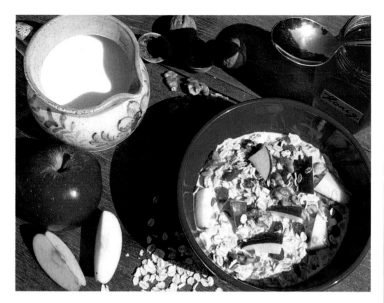

The muesli recipe by Dr. Max Bircher-Brenner is based on a healthful mixture of yogurt, oats, fruit, and nuts (for recipe, see page 82). You will give your body an optimal start in the morning with this muesli.

Hildegard von Bingen's Pear Honey

According to Abbess Hildegard von Bingen, pear honey is the best means of purification you can use.

Why don't you try the recipe (in the sidebar)? It is supposed to be especially good for headaches, migraines, and troubled breathing. To conduct the cure, it's important to eat the honey daily for at least two to three months. This is the procedure:

➤ One teaspoon in the morning on an empty stomach
➤ Two teaspoons at noon, after lunch
➤ One teaspoon at night before going to sleep

Possible Combinations

Depending on your preference, you can stay on a cure for a week or a few days. You can even combine the following:

➤ Pear honey and Bircher muesli
➤ Dandelion salad and vegetable soup
➤ Lime blossom tea and potatoes stuffed with quark
➤ A cure with whey and a raw food plate

Vegetable Broth
Ingredients
Half an onion with skin, 2 parsley roots, 1 small celery root, ½ cabbage, 2 small leeks, a few leaves of mangel-wurzel, 1 bay leaf, 1 pinch of dried basil.

Preparation
Wash the vegetables, cut, and place in 2 liters (or qt.) of cold water. Add bay leaf and basil, and simmer for 2 hours on low heat. Then strain. Rice can be cooked in the broth.

A Mild Purification Cure, by Dr. Erich Rauch

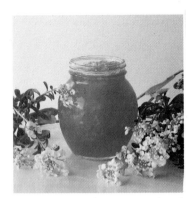

Honey not only is a natural and delicious sweetener, but it also is good for you.

This mild purification cure can be used on normal working days. It is important that you chew well over the course of this cure.

This is a very gentle cleansing diet that aims to unburden and regenerate stressed intestines. Furthermore, with this diet, the acid-base balance is restored. The cure was devised by Dr. Erich Rauch, a pupil of Dr. F. X. Mayr, inventor of the milk roll cure mentioned earlier.

This mild purification is especially recommended for working people, as it can be used during normal working days. It also can be conducted over a longer period of time than other cures and under stressful conditions.

On this diet, you will eat three times a day (no in-between meals) small portions of food that is of high biological quality and easy to digest. Avoid fatty food and food high in cellulose, because they are hard to digest, induce flatulence, and are heavy. For every meal, eat only until you feel slightly satiated.

Just as with the milk roll cure, great emphasis is placed on chewing every single bite of food for a long time (at least 30 times); thus the food is best prepared for entering the digestive system and you will be satiated sooner.

By referring to the following lists, you can design your own meals. This dietary cure contains all vital foods and minerals, and you can continue it for several weeks without worrying about food deficiencies.

What You May Eat on the Diet

➤ Plant-based oils: Cold-pressed, highly saturated fatty acids, some butter, plant-based margarine
➤ For sweetening: Thickened juice of pears, maple syrup, honey, yogurt, buttermilk, low-fat quark, kefir, low-fat cheeses, etc.
➤ Vegetables: Cooked (for example, carrots, celery, parsley, black daikon, broccoli, spinach, fennel, red beets, tomatoes, zucchini) and as a soup, also potatoes in their skin
➤ Eggs: Soft boiled
➤ Fish, poultry, and meat: Lean varieties (fowl, veal, beef, trout) steamed or grilled, but no more than twice a week
➤ Grain: Easily digestible (for example, oats, millet, rice, and buckwheat), plus unsweetened cornflakes, semolina, aged rolls (cure rolls)
➤ Beverages: Mineral water and herbal teas (2 to 3 liters, or quarts), malt coffee
➤ Spices: Sea salt, fresh herbs, yeast flakes

On the opposite lists, you will find foods that you can eat or should avoid during the cure.

What You Should Avoid

➤ Foods rich in cellulose: Fresh, rich, whole-kernel breads, and dishes made with kale, cabbage, and legumes
➤ Raw food: Fresh fruit and vegetables, salads because they ferment so strongly in the intestines, plus sweet sauces, fruit juices, and all canned fruit
➤ Fatty foods: Pork, all sausages because they contain a lot of fat and pork, gravies, mayonnaise, animal fats like lard
➤ White flour and refined sugar: All sweets, marmalades, torts, custards, baked goods, and yeast pastries
➤ Drugs: Alcohol, nicotine, coffee (except for decaffeinated), soft drinks

Designing Your Personal Diet Plan

"The intestines go to sleep with the chickens and get up with them."—F. X. Mayr

Of the three meals you are allowed per day, the evening meal should be the smallest. You would unburden your intestines further if you were to skip the evening meal altogether once in a while and only drink 2 cups of herbal tea sweetened with honey. This would be in line with the time when the digestive system has its natural rest.

Supplementary Measures

If you stick to the four basic rules for eating correctly, you will see that you will be able to taste food more intensely and you will be satiated sooner.

Eat cure rolls as often as possible. You are already familiar with then from the Mayr cure on page 67. A cure roll is a wheat roll that has been left to dry out in the open for about three days. As an additional detoxification measure, Dr. Rauch recommends taking a torso-rub bath (see page 94) every day or two during the mild purification cure.

How to Eat Correctly

Please follow these guidelines:
➤ Take only small bites into your mouth.
➤ Chew all food for a long time to produce saliva.
➤ Enjoy every bite.
➤ Stop eating as soon as you feel slightly satiated.

Suggested Daily Schedule

➤ *After rising:* Glauber or Epsom-salts solution to clean the intestines (about every two days), dry-brush massage, hot-and-cold shower.

➤ *Breakfast:* Milk, malt coffee, or herbal tea with teaspoon of honey, a cure roll with butter, a soft-boiled egg or some quark.

➤ Or oatmeal: Add 3 tablespoons of oats to ¼ liter (or quart) of boiling water, and continue to boil for 2 minutes. Stir in ⅛ liter of milk, simmer for 2 minutes, and strain.

➤ *Before lunch*: Rest for 30 minutes with a hot-water bottle.

➤ *Lunch:* Vegetable broth (see page 89), cooked vegetables, some grilled fish or meat, potatoes in their skin,

quark with fruit.

➤ Or: Thick potato-vegetable soup (page 31), potatoes in their skin with a little butter, and salt, grilled fish.

➤ Or: Raw high-quality ground meat mixed with the yolk of an egg, onions, pepper, paprika, a little salt and capers, and crisp bread.

➤ *Afternoon:* An hour of physical exercise in fresh air.

➤ *Evening:* Two cups of herbal tea (for example, mint, mallow, wild agrimony) with a teaspoon of honey, a cure roll, some low-fat cheese.

➤ *Later:* Dry-brush massage or torso-rub bath, go to bed early, put a hot-water bottle or a liver wrap on your stomach.

Today, with higher and higher costs for hospital care, and more and more medications being prescribed, isn't it time to try naturopathic healing?

A Plea for Natural Treatment

"If more and more hospitals and more and more physicians are needed, then this fact cries out for a basic treatment for the ills produced by affluence and abundance or overabundance." —Dr. Erich Rauch, Director of the Mayr Cure Clinic in Maria Wörth-Dellach, Austria

Torso-Rub Bath, by Louis Kuhne

The torso-rub bath devised by Louis Kuhne (1835–1901) is an excellent measure to accelerate detoxification via all organs of elimination. You will need a sitz bath, in which you can sit down relaxed and be able to lean back; your feet and lower legs should rest on a stool and not get wet. The water in the tub should reach up to your navel.

How to Take the Torso-Rub Bath

➤ Sit down in the bath as described (it is best to wear woolen socks on your feet). Depending on your preference, the water temperature should be between 20 and 28°C (68 and 82°F), but the cooler the better. Add the cold water slowly. Increase the length of the bath gradually, from 5 to 7 minutes to 15 to 20 minutes, and stay in until your body is cooled down.

➤ Over the duration of the bath, without stopping once, rub your abdomen from the navel downward with a rough washcloth. Rub the lower abdomen in a crisscross fashion especially well. The pubic area, is massaged too; then the abdomen is massaged again.

➤ Climb out of the tub, and rub yourself down with a rough bath towel. It is important to warm up quickly after the bath. During the summer, take a sunbath, jog, or do another kind of physical activity. Otherwise, take a hot shower, put a hot-water bottle on your stomach, put on warm socks and a heavy bathrobe, and/or drink hot herbal tea. If you take this bath frequently, you will find that you will feel nicely warm from the inside without having to do much of anything afterward.

➤ You can take the torso-rub bath once a day.

➤ Do not take the bath right after a meal.

The torso-rub bath aids all functions of the digestive system, supports the cleansing work of the kidneys, invigorates breathing and the skin, and improves blood circulation.

TIP

As an alternative to a sitz tub, you also can use a plastic bathtub for children, which you can place in your own bathtub.

Index

About the Authors

MARGOT HELMISS is a journalist. Her main fields of interest are methods of natural healing and alternative therapies.

FALK SCHREITHAUER is a writer and journalist working in the areas of man, nature, and health.

Picture Credits

AKG, Berlin: 28, 86; Bavaria, Gauting: front cover; IFA-Bilderteam, Taufkirchen: 33 (Digul), 39 (Diaf), 46 (Lederer), 62, 65 (Schmitz), 69 (Eich); Alfred Pasieka, Hilden: 17; Premium, Dusseldorf: 23 (Orion Press); The Image Bank: 1 (H.Wolf), 5 (Jeff Hunter), 53 (Eliane Sulle); Tony Stone, Munich: 6 (Terry Vine), 76 (Dan Bosler); Transglobe Agency, Hamburg: 13, 60 (Jerrican), 74 (Trizep), 89 (Zone 5), 90 (Jo Clasen)